Somatics

A Comprehensive Guide to Somatic Therapy Workouts for Stress Relief

(A Step-by-step Guide to Reclaiming Your Body)

Joseph Portis

Published By **Darby Connor**

Joseph Portis

Somatics: A Comprehensive Guide to Somatic Therapy Workouts for Stress Relief (A Step-by-step Guide to Reclaiming Your Body)

ISBN 978-1-9995143-4-1

Legal & Disclaimer

Table Of Contents

Chapter 1: Foundations Of Somatic Therapy

What is Somatic Therapy?

Somatic therapy, additionally referred to as somatic experiencing remedy, is a restoration modality designed to deal with PTSD and numerous highbrow and emotional wellbeing worries via fostering a profound connection between the mind and frame. This technique places a strong emphasis on the body, facilitating the discharge of strain, anxiety, and trauma held inside the physical self.

In assessment to conventional intellectual fitness strategies like CBT, which extra frequently than no longer target the mind, somatic treatment integrates body targeted strategies like dance, breathe work, and meditation to facilitate emotional healing. Moreover, somatic experiencing treatment combines verbal treatment with bodily video games that bridge the distance a number of the thoughts and the body.

Types of Somatic Therapy

Somatic therapy, frequently known as somatic experiencing treatment, represents one of the maximum installed and direct strategies within the realm of healing practices. Unlike traditional mental wellness treatments that at the entire encompass verbal communication, somatic remedy encourages patients to delve into their troubles thru centering their attention on their underlying physical sensations. Within this recovery framework, masses of thoughts body physical games are employed, which encompass breath work, meditation, visualization, massage, grounding strategies, dance, and heightened sensory consciousness.

Furthermore, somatic therapy's versatility extends beyond its critical form. Several specialized subgroups have followed its framework to tailor their techniques in brilliant methods. These subgroups include:

1. Sensor motor psychotherapy: An all encompassing healing technique that harnesses the body as a wealthy deliver of insights and as a purpose for intervention.

2. The Hakomi Method: A psychotherapeutic exercise that harmoniously integrates scientific, highbrow, and religious perspectives, centering on 4 fundamental standards: gentleness, nonviolence, compassion, and mindfulness.

three. Bioenergetic assessment: A form of bodytargeted psychotherapy that amalgamates bodily, analytical, and relational strategies, based on the facts of power dynamics.

four. Biodynamic psychotherapy: A holistic treatment technique that blends conventional scientific strategies with opportunity recuperation modalities, which consist of fingerson rub down administered with the resource of the therapist.

5. Brainspotting: Beyond traditional communicate therapy, this modality consists of the region of the eyes to rewire emotional responses, complementing thoughts and bodyoriented strategies.

Techniques

Somatic treatment is grounded inside the notion that lifestyles opinions are not entirely restricted to the mind however are also imprinted within the frame. This healing approach adopts a holistic perspective, addressing each the bodily sensations inside your body and open communicate about your worrying conditions. Within the area of somatic therapy, a numerous array of strategies is employed, which includes:

1. Cultivating heightened popularity of bodily sensations.

2. Harnessing your emotional reservoirs.

three. Establishing a experience of grounding.

4. Encouraging complex verbal descriptions.

4

5. Incorporating physical movements, together with the expression of physical sensations.

6. Equipping oneself with equipment for emotional regulation.

7. Shifting focus amongst worrying and nondemanding factors to facilitate tension release.

eight. Revisiting beyond conditions with newfound physical strategies.

9. Facilitating emotional release.

10. Fortifying private boundaries.

What Somatic Therapy Can Help With?

Somatic Therapy's Versatility in Addressing Challenges

Somatic remedy is a flexible approach that offers an opportunity to standard speak therapy. It is executed to a wide range of every intellectual and bodily health concerns.

In the realm of intellectual fitness, somatic therapy has showed effectiveness in addressing:

1. PostTraumatic Stress Disorder (PTSD)

2. Anxiety

three. Addiction

four. Grief

five. Depression

6. Stress

On the bodily the the front, somatic therapy may be useful for individuals coping with:

1. Chronic ache

2. Digestive troubles

three. Sexual disorder

Due to its emphasis on grounding and mindfulness, somatic treatment proves to be a valuable opportunity for those looking for a deeper connection with themselves and a more profound knowledge of their existence reviews.

Factors to Ponder

When embarking on any recuperation adventure, it is critical to be emotionally and mentally prepared, with enough time and energy to delve into complex feelings. If you pick inman or woman somatic treatment, bodily contact is frequently part of the approach, necessitating a consolation degree with such interactions.

Maintaining smooth barriers and acquiring consent are paramount when it comes to tactile factors of remedy. Rest confident, you will by no means experience any bodily contact without your specific consent.

It is in truth well really worth noting that somatic remedy is commonly seemed as a stable form of therapy with out a great or one among a type risks associated with its technique.

The Origins of Somatic Therapy

Somatic remedy, regularly called somatic experiencing or somatic psychology, has its roots in severa fields, which includes psychology, neuroscience, and bodycentered practices. This segment will discover the historic and theoretical foundations of somatic therapy, losing moderate at the manner it advanced into the effective healing modality it's far in recent times.

Historical Background

Somatic remedy draws idea from ancient healing practices that identified the profound connection some of the thoughts and the frame. Indigenous cultures and ancient Eastern traditions, which includes yoga, Tai Chi, and mindfulness meditation, have lengthy understood the significance of somatic cognizance and the position it performs in conventional wellbeing. These traditions emphasised the significance of staying observed in one's body to gain intellectual, emotional, and bodily concord.

However, the modern development of somatic therapy owes plenty to the pioneering paintings of several key figures:

Wilhelm Reich (18971957): A psychoanalyst and psychiatrist, Reich made huge contributions to the expertise of the mindframe connection. He introduced the idea of "body armor," which recommended that emotional trauma should seem as bodily anxiety and anxiety in the body. Reich's art work laid the basis for somatic treatment thru highlighting the bodily manifestations of emotional pain.

Moshe Feldenkrais (19041984): Feldenkrais have become an Israeli physicist and engineer who developed the Feldenkrais Method. This technique specializes in improving bodily and emotional wellbeing via recognition of motion and posture. The Feldenkrais Method has been instrumental within the development of somatic therapy strategies.

Alexander Lowen (19102008): A student of Wilhelm Reich, Lowen extended on Reich's mind and advanced Bioenergetic Analysis, a form of somatic remedy that emphasizes the release of emotional and bodily anxiety thru breath, motion, and selfpopularity.

Thomas Hanna (19281990): Hanna's paintings on Somatics delivered the concept that habitual forms of muscular anxiety is probably modified thru aware attention and movement. This concept is foundational to many somatic treatment practices.

Contemporary Approaches

Today, somatic remedy has superior right proper right into a diverse region encompassing numerous strategies, at the side of Somatic Experiencing (superior through manner of Peter A. Levine), Sensorimotor Psychotherapy (evolved via Pat Ogden), and Hakomi Therapy (advanced thru Ron Kurtz), amongst others. These present day processes have included elements from psychology, neuroscience, and frametargeted treatment options to create powerful strategies for healing trauma and selling everyday nicelybeing.

At the coronary coronary coronary heart of somatic remedy lies the important principle that the body shops and shows emotional reviews. By developing somatic cognizance—turning into attuned to bodily sensations, emotions, and actions—you can advantage belief into beyond traumas and paintings in the course of resolving them. Somatic remedy emphasizes the importance of present2d enjoy, encouraging individuals to reconnect with their our bodies and explore the understanding held inner.

As we delve deeper into this ebook, we are able to discover how somatic remedy techniques are finished in exercise to help human beings heal from trauma, lessen pressure, and domesticate a stronger mindbody connection. Understanding the origins of somatic remedy offers treasured context for appreciating its transformative capability.

Core Principles of Somatic Therapy

Somatic Therapy is based on severa middle ideas that guide its exercising and effectiveness. Understanding the ones principles is crucial for anyone searching out to embark on a journey of recuperation and selfdiscovery via this modality. In this phase, we can discover the critical standards of Somatic Therapy:

1. The Body Holds Wisdom: Somatic Therapy operates on the perception that the body holds a reservoir of knowledge and statistics about our studies, specially demanding ones. It acknowledges that our our bodies do not forget what our minds could probable overlook about, and by way of tuning into bodily sensations, we are capable of get proper of entry to this saved facts.

2. MindBody Connection: At the coronary coronary heart of Somatic Therapy is the concept of the mindframe connection. It acknowledges that our intellectual and emotional states are intricately related to our

bodily sensations. Trauma can show up as tension, ache, or discomfort in the body, and conversely, calming the body may additionally have a calming impact on the thoughts.

3. Safety and Titration: Safety is paramount in Somatic Therapy. It emphasizes that recuperation must hold at a pace snug for the person. The method of titration consists of taking small, practicable steps in addressing trauma to save you overwhelming emotional responses. This precept guarantees that recuperation is moderate and sustainable.

4. Awareness and Presence: Somatic Therapy encourages heightened selfinterest and presence within the 2nd. Practitioners are taught to check physical sensations with out judgment, bearing in mind a deep knowhow of their emotional states. This cognizance is a cornerstone of recovery.

5. Embodiment: Embodiment refers to the exercising of clearly inhabiting one's body and being gift within the bodily experience. This precept emphasizes that recuperation takes

vicinity thru a felt experience of the frame, in place of definitely via highbrow understanding. It encourages human beings to reconnect with their our our bodies and keep in thoughts their bodily sensations.

6. Release and Integration: Somatic Therapy focuses on freeing saved trauma and integrating fragmented elements of the self. It recognizes that unresolved trauma can result in disconnection from factors of oneself and objectives to facilitate the reintegration of those additives right right into a cohesive whole.

7. Holistic Approach: Somatic Therapy takes a holistic method to recuperation, recognizing that people are complex beings inspired via their surroundings, relationships, and way of lifestyles. It considers the ones sorts of factors in the restoration way, promoting no longer in truth symptom remedy but average properlybeing and personal increase.

Chapter 2: The Science Of Trauma And The Body

Trauma and the Nervous System

When an man or woman undergoes a traumatic event, their sympathetic nervous machine becomes engaged, essential to the discharge of stress hormones collectively with cortisol and adrenaline. These hormonal responses increase heart charge, boom blood pressure, and accelerate respiratory, all of which serve to put together the body for both confronting or escaping from a perceived chance.

The Autonomic Nervous System

The autonomic worried device (ANS) is a vital problem of our physiological makeup that plays a treasured role in how our our bodies respond to strain, chance, and ordinary situations. Understanding the ANS is critical at the same time as delving into the technology of trauma and its effects at the body.

Anatomy of the Autonomic Nervous System

The ANS is split into two important branches, every chargeable for distinct physiological responses:

Sympathetic Nervous System (SNS): Often known as the "fight or flight" machine, the SNS prepares the body to answer to perceived threats. It triggers the discharge of pressure hormones like adrenaline, will boom coronary heart price, and redirects blood glide far from nonvital abilties, such as digestion, closer to muscle companies and organs desired for fast movement.

Parasympathetic Nervous System (PNS): The PNS is the body's "rest and digest" device. It promotes rest, slows the coronary coronary heart charge, and permits the frame to hold electricity. This branch is answerable for returning the body to a state of equilibrium after the SNS has been activated.

The Role of the ANS in Trauma

Trauma has a profound impact on the functioning of the autonomic involved system. When an person memories a demanding event, the ANS reaction can grow to be dysregulated, essential to numerous bodily and emotional signs and symptoms and signs and signs:

Hypervigilance: Trauma can go away the SNS in a heightened u . S . Of alertness, causing human beings to be overly touchy to capability threats of their surroundings. This can motive chronic stress and anxiety.

Hyperarousal: The persistent activation of the SNS can bring about signs together with increased heart fee, shallow breathing, and muscle tension, contributing to feelings of panic and agitation.

Hypoarousal: On the opposite hand, a few trauma survivors enjoy a state of hypoarousal, wherein the PNS dominance outcomes in emotions of numbness, dissociation, and emotional detachment.

Polyvagal Theory

To further apprehend the complexities of the autonomic concerned gadget's reaction to trauma, it's far crucial to discover the Polyvagal Theory developed thru Dr. Stephen Porges. This precept sheds light on how the ANS operates in social engagement, combat or flight, and shutdown modes, imparting insights into how trauma influences our capability to hook up with others and alter our emotions.

Healing the ANS Through Somatic Therapy

One of the vital dreams of somatic remedy is to restore balance to the autonomic annoying gadget. This section will introduce readers to numerous somatic techniques and sporting occasions designed to assist human beings adjust their ANS, reduce stress, and cope with traumaassociated signs and symptoms and signs and symptoms.

Breathing Exercises: Explore precise respiration techniques that interact the PNS, promoting rest and emotional regulation.

Body Awareness Practices: Learn how somatic remedy encourages human beings to track into bodily sensations to choose out and launch stored trauma.

Movement and Embodiment: Understand the function of physical motion and bodily sports in reestablishing a healthful ANS reaction.

Mindfulness and Meditation: Discover mindfulness practices which could assist people stay grounded and gift, lowering the reactivity of the ANS.

The Role of the Brain in Trauma

The human thoughts is an hard and powerful organ, and it performs a relevant position in how we experience and reply to trauma. Understanding the brain's involvement in trauma can offer treasured insights into the often complicated and prolongedlasting effects of annoying evaluations.

The Triune Brain Model

To understand the thoughts's characteristic in trauma, it is beneficial to keep in mind the triune mind version. This version, proposed with the resource of using American neuroscientist and psychiatrist Paul D. MacLean, divides the thoughts into 3 remarkable components, each associated with wonderful abilties and evolutionary tiers.

1. Reptilian Brain (The Brainstem): This is the most primitive part of the thoughts, accountable for number one survival capabilities including breathing, coronary coronary heart price law, and fightorflight responses. When a worrying event takes area, the brainstem reacts almost straight away thru triggering the release of strain hormones like adrenaline, getting prepared the body for instant movement.

2. Mammalian Brain (The Limbic System): The limbic system, which includes structures similar to the amygdala and hippocampus, is associated with emotions, memory formation, and social bonding. In trauma, the amygdala,

in particular, can become hypersensitive, foremost to heightened emotional responses, mainly fear and tension. Traumatic memories can also additionally emerge as deeply ingrained in the hippocampus, contributing to flashbacks and intrusive mind.

three. Human Brain (The Neocortex): The neocortex, the most currently advanced part of the mind, is chargeable for betterorder questioning, desiremaking, and reasoning. In the context of trauma, this a part of the thoughts can battle to make enjoy of the overwhelming emotions and physical sensations, often essential to cognitive distortions, guilt, and selfblame.

Neuroplasticity and Trauma

One of the reSolomonable factors of the mind is its ability for neuroplasticity. This refers to the mind's capability to reorganize itself by way of way of forming new neural connections all through lifestyles. In the context of trauma, neuroplasticity can work every for and within the direction of healing.

Maladaptive Plasticity: Traumatic tales can result in maladaptive adjustments in the brain's shape and function. This can result in persistent strain, emotional dysregulation, and the development of traumaassociated problems like PTSD.

Adaptive Plasticity: On the high excellent side, the mind can also adapt in strategies that sell healing. With the right interventions and healing techniques, it's far viable to rewire the brain, steadily decreasing the effect of demanding recollections and signs and symptoms.

The Prefrontal Cortex and Trauma

The prefrontal cortex, a part of the human mind's neocortex, performs a critical position in regulating emotions and making rational decisions. However, trauma can disrupt the functioning of this region. Individuals who have skilled trauma regularly discover it difficult to regulate their emotions successfully. They might also moreover struggle with impulse manage and find out it difficult to make choices with out being overwhelmed through the usage of worry or anxiety.

Understanding the feature of the mind in trauma is crucial for each humans attempting to find restoration and the professionals who help them. It highlights the complex interplay amongst physiological responses, emotional reactions, and cognitive techniques, all of which have to be considered in the journey inside the path of recovery.

How Trauma Impacts the Body

Trauma isn't always absolutely an occasion that occurs in the mind; it leaves a longlasting imprint at the frame as nicely. Understanding how trauma affects the body is a vital step in the journey inside the course of healing and recuperation. When worrying testimonies get up, the body goes via a complex series of physiological responses which could have profound and lasting effects. In this section, we'll discover the ones influences in detail.

The Stress Response System

Trauma activates the body's pressure response device, frequently called the "fight or flight" response. This device is designed to assist us react quick in risky conditions, however at the same time as it's far caused by using the usage of trauma, it is able to have unfavourable effects. Key elements of the strain response system embody:

1. Release of Stress Hormones: The thoughts alerts the discharge of pressure hormones like cortisol and adrenaline. These hormones put together the frame for movement, developing coronary coronary coronary heart fee, blood stress, and application.

2. Heightened Arousal: Trauma can bring about a continual kingdom of heightened arousal. Survivors can also moreover emerge as hypervigilant, constantly scanning their surroundings for threats, even in secure conditions.

3. Impaired Memory: The stress response can impair reminiscence competencies. Traumatic recollections may be fragmented or tough to hold in thoughts, that would make a contribution to feelings of false impression and helplessness.

The Impact on the Nervous System

The fearful tool performs a crucial feature in how the body responds to trauma. It includes number one branches:

1. Sympathetic Nervous System (SNS): This branch of the nerveracking device is responsible for the "combat or flight" reaction. It revs up the body's energy for fast motion.

2. Parasympathetic Nervous System (PNS): The PNS is answerable for rest and recovery. It helps the frame cross lower back to a country of calm after a risk has handed.

Trauma disrupts the stability the various ones structures. Survivors regularly locate themselves stuck in a country of sympathetic dominance, unable to loosen up and get better absolutely. This chronic activation can result in some of physical signs and symptoms and signs and symptoms, together with:

Chronic Muscle Tension: Continuous stress can cause muscular tissues to live traumatic, fundamental to aches and pains, particularly within the neck, shoulders, and back.

Digestive Problems: The digestive device can also come to be impaired, resulting in problems like irritable bowel syndrome (IBS) or persistent indigestion.

Sleep Disturbances: Trauma can disrupt sleep patterns, fundamental to insomnia, nightmares, or harassed sleep.

Immune System Dysfunction: Prolonged strain weakens the immune device, making the frame extra vulnerable to contamination.

Cardiovascular Issues: Longterm stress can make a contribution to excessive blood strain and an expanded hazard of coronary coronary heart illness.

The MindBody Feedback Loop

One of the most fascinating elements of trauma's effect on the body is the mindbody comments loop. Traumatic stories can purpose a constant cycle of physical sensations, feelings, and mind:

Physical Sensations: Trauma survivors often experience physical signs and symptoms and symptoms and symptoms which encompass speedy heartbeat, shallow respiration, or muscle anxiety, even though there may be no instant hazard.

Emotional Distress: These physical sensations can trigger excessive emotions like worry, tension, or anger.

Cognitive Responses: In reaction to the ones feelings, survivors may additionally moreover have distorted or horrible thoughts approximately themselves, their safety, or their future.

Understanding this comments loop is crucial as it approach that recovery trauma isn't always pretty a whole lot addressing the mind or the frame in isolation. It's about spotting and interrupting this cycle to repair stability and nicelybeing.

Chapter 3: Unearthing The Trauma

Recognizing Trauma Symptoms

Recognizing trauma signs and symptoms is a essential step at the direction to healing. Trauma regularly leaves a profound impact on an character's bodily, emotional, and intellectual properlybeing. In this chapter, we will explore the common signs of trauma, the techniques wherein it could take region in each day existence, and the importance of selfpopularity on this system.

Common Symptoms of Trauma

Trauma may additionally have an impact on people in severa tactics, and its signs can also additionally variety from character to individual. However, there are several commonplace signs and symptoms and symptoms and signs and symptoms and symptoms to be aware about:

1. Flashbacks and Intrusive Memories: Trauma survivors can also experience superb and distressing flashbacks of the disturbing

occasion. These memories may be added approximately thru using seemingly unrelated stimuli.

2. Avoidance Behaviors: People often visit exquisite lengths to keep away from conditions, locations, or people that remind them of the trauma. This can motive social isolation and restricted life reviews.

three. Hyperarousal: Individuals with trauma can be in a regular kingdom of alertness, feeling effortlessly startled, irritable, or stressful. They may have trouble dozing and enjoy a heightened startle response.

4. Emotional Numbing: Some trauma survivors enjoy emotional numbness. They also can discover it tough to connect with their personal feelings or the emotions of others.

5. Negative Changes in Thinking and Mood: This includes persistent horrible thoughts, selfblame, guilt, and a experience of hopelessness. Depression and tension

disorders are commonplace cooccurring conditions.

The Longterm Effects of Unaddressed Trauma

Understanding the lengthytime period results of unaddressed trauma is important for people in search of restoration. Unresolved trauma can purpose:

1. Chronic Health Issues: Trauma is connected to a number of bodily fitness issues, which includes continual ache, coronary coronary heart sickness, and autoimmune issues.

2. Substance Abuse: Some people flip to pills or alcohol as a way to deal with trauma signs, that could motive dependancy problems.

three. Relationship Problems: Trauma can pressure relationships, fundamental to problems in forming and retaining connections with others.

four. Impaired Work and Academic Performance: Trauma could have an impact on one's ability to concentrate, ensuing in disturbing conditions at art work or in school.

The Importance of Selfattention

Selfinterest is the cornerstone of spotting trauma signs and symptoms and signs. It entails being in song collectively with your emotions, physical sensations, and concept patterns. Here's why it subjects:

1. Early Intervention: Recognizing signs and symptoms and symptoms early lets in for nicely timed intervention and get right of entry to to suitable help systems.

2. Empowerment: Understanding that your struggles may be associated with trauma can empower you to take steps inside the route of healing and are looking for expert assist.

3. Reducing SelfBlame: Selfpopularity permits humans recognize that trauma signs and symptoms are a natural reaction to an unusual occasion and no longer a sign of private susceptible factor or failure.

4. Choice: With selfhobby, you gain the ability to pick the manner you reply to trauma signs and signs, in place of being controlled by way of way of them.

In the journey in the direction of recovery, spotting trauma symptoms is step one. It's a courageous acknowledgment of your testimonies and the start of a course closer to restoration. In the subsequent chapters, we are able to find out techniques and strategies to address the ones symptoms and regain manage over your existence.

Chapter 4: The Mind Body Connection

Understanding the Mind Body Connection

The thoughts and body are in element linked, and this profound dating performs a pivotal function inside the experience of trauma and its recuperation. In this financial wreck, we delve deeper into the complex net that binds our thoughts, emotions, and bodily sensations. By gaining belief. into this connection, you'll be better prepared to navigate the course inside the course of recovery and wellbeing.

The BrainBody Link

In the tough net of human life, the brain and body are inseparable partners. They talk in a complex dance, converting statistics, feelings, and reactions. This interconnectedness paperwork the foundation of somatic remedy's effectiveness in recovery trauma and nurturing the thoughtsbody connection.

Understanding the BrainBody Connection

At the middle of the brainbody hyperlink lies the nervous system, an complicated network responsible for transmitting information at a few level inside the frame. Two key components of the nerveracking device play pivotal roles in facts this connection: the crucial anxious gadget (CNS) and the peripheral nervous device (PNS).

1. Central Nervous System (CNS): This consists of the mind and spinal wire. It serves due to the fact the command center, processing facts and coordinating responses. The mind, specifically, is a reSolomonable organ that not simplest regulates physical abilities however moreover shops reminiscences, techniques feelings, and governs our cognitive capabilities.

2. Peripheral Nervous System (PNS): The PNS extends past the CNS, carrying out out to each part of the frame. It's responsible for transmitting sensory information to the mind and sporting out motor instructions. This system is split into branches: the somatic

apprehensive device, which controls voluntary actions, and the autonomic nervous device (ANS), which manages involuntary features like coronary heart charge and digestion.

Emotions and the Body

Emotions aren't certainly precis emotions experienced inside the thoughts; they are deeply intertwined with the frame's bodily sensations. When you experience pride, your frame might in all likelihood respond with a warmth, open chest and a lightness in the doorstep. Conversely, whilst you revel in worry, your frame might probable disturbing up, your coronary coronary heart price speeds up, and your muscle tissues put together for movement.

1. The Emotional Blueprint: Emotions are hardwired into our biology. They have superior as adaptive responses to numerous situations. For instance, worry triggers a "combat or flight" response, getting ready the body to confront hazard or escape it. This

immediately physical response to emotional stimuli is a testomony to the profound link amongst our minds and our our bodies.

2. Emotional Memory: The mind now not fine strategies emotions but additionally shops them as reminiscences. Traumatic critiques can depart imprints in our neural pathways, main to bodily reactions although the emotional cause is not present. These emotional reminiscences can make a contribution to signs of trauma.

The Body's Wisdom

One of the fundamental requirements of somatic remedy is spotting that the frame holds its personal knowledge. It remembers past reviews, each fine and horrible, and it communicates its needs through physical sensations and symptoms. Tuning into this bodily knowledge is important for recuperation trauma and fostering emotional nicelybeing.

1. Physical Sensations as Messengers: When we experience ache or pain in our our our our bodies, it's often a signal that some thing needs interest. These sensations may be messages from our subconscious, telling us in which healing is needed. Somatic remedy encourages us to pay attention to and interpret those alerts.

2. Unblocking Energy: Trauma and stress can create blockages within the frame's electricity flow, maximum crucial to bodily and emotional pain. Techniques in somatic remedy cause to release those blockages, restoring stability and concord to each thoughts and body.

By facts the mindbody connection, we benefit perception into how trauma influences us on a physiological degree and the way somatic therapy can assist us release the body's innate functionality for recuperation.

Emotions and Physical Sensations

In the adventure of recovery trauma via somatic remedy, it is important to understand the intimate courting among our feelings and physical sensations. This connection regularly goes omitted in our each day lives, but it performs a pivotal characteristic in each the enjoy of trauma and its selection. In this phase, we are able to discover how feelings occur inside the body and the way spotting those bodily sensations may be a effective tool for recuperation.

The Embodied Nature of Emotions

Emotions aren't in fact precis feelings that arise in our minds; they're deeply rooted in our bodies. When you experience unhappiness, joy, fear, anger, or some other emotion, your body responds in various strategies. These bodily responses can include changes in coronary coronary heart price, muscle tension, respiration styles, or even digestion. Here's a higher take a look at how some not unusual emotions show up in the frame:

Sadness: Often skilled as a heaviness in the chest, a lump inside the throat, or a sensation of sinking.

Joy: Can show up as lightness, a enjoy of expansion, or a heat and open feeling inside the chest and coronary coronary coronary heart area.

Fear: Typically accompanied thru way of a racing coronary coronary heart, shallow respiratory, muscle anxiety, and a sense of tightness or constriction.

Anger: May motive extended coronary heart charge, clenched fists, increased frame temperature, and a surge of strength.

The Body's Memory of Emotions

One of the reSolomonable factors of somatic remedy is that our our bodies recollect past emotional studies, specially demanding ones. Even prolonged after the demanding event has passed off, the body can preserve onto the bodily sensations associated with that trauma. This is why people who have skilled trauma often report feeling added about through reputedly unrelated activities that evoke a bodily memory of the trauma.

Understanding this connection amongst feelings and bodily sensations is a important part of somatic therapy. By turning into aware of how your frame responds to important emotions, you can begin to recognize patterns and triggers related to past traumas.

Exploring Your Own EmotionBody Connection

To harness the strength of the emotionframe connection, it's far essential to exercise selfcognizance and mindfulness. Here's a smooth exercise you could try:

1. Find a quiet and cushty area to sit down or lie down.

2. Close your eyes and take a few deep breaths to center yourself.

3. Begin to check your body from head to toe, paying near attention to any bodily sensations.

4. As you do this, bring to thoughts numerous emotions. Start with a independent emotion like happiness and then progress to more complex ones like disappointment or anger.

five. Notice how your body responds to every emotion. Are there areas of hysteria, relaxation, warmth, or pain?

6. Don't determine or try to alternate these sensations; actually take a look at them without attachment.

This exercise assist you to turn out to be greater in track along with your emotionframe connection. It's an essential step inside the somatic remedy technique because it allows you to find out and launch saved feelings and physical tension, in the end contributing for your recovery adventure.

How Emotions Manifest in the Body

Understanding how emotions arise within the body is a essential factor of somatic remedy. Emotions are not summary thoughts confined to the mind; they've got a profound impact on the body, and this thoughtsframe connection performs a important characteristic in trauma and healing. In this phase, we discover how awesome emotions can take area physically and why this popularity is crucial to your recuperation adventure.

1. The Body due to the reality the Emotional Canvas

Our our bodies are like canvases in which feelings paint vivid photographs. Every emotion, whether or not or not extraordinary or negative, triggers a very specific set of bodily responses. These responses may be subtle or extreme, counting on the emotional depth. Here are a few not unusual approaches feelings take vicinity inside the body:

Anxiety: Anxiety frequently gives as a racing coronary coronary heart, shallow breathing, muscle tension (especially within the shoulders and neck), and a knot within the stomach. These bodily sensations are a part of the body's "combat or flight" reaction.

Sadness: When we're sad, we'd experience heaviness in our chest, tears welling up in our eyes, and a droop in our posture. This bodily manifestation of unhappiness is why it's far regularly described as a "heavy" emotion.

Joy: Joy is related to a lightness within the body. You ought to possibly word a skip inside the doorstep, a grin for your face, and a enjoy of energy and energy whilst you revel in pleasure.

Anger: Anger tends to create a surge of power in the frame. You may additionally clench your fists, grind your enamel, or revel in your face flush. This bodily reaction is part of the frame's education for motion.

Chapter 5: Somatic Techniques For Healing

Grounding and Centering Techniques

In the previous chapters, we explored the profound connection amongst trauma, the mind, and the frame. Now, it's time to delve into practical tools that permit you to regain manipulate over your body and feelings. Grounding and centering techniques are the muse of somatic therapy, serving as powerful anchors to the prevailing 2nd and a way to reconnect collectively collectively along with your frame's innate consciousness.

Breathwork and Mindfulness

Your breath is an great pleasant pal to your recuperation adventure. It's a bridge amongst your aware thoughts and your frame's autonomic abilities. By training conscious respiratory, you can modify your concerned gadget, lessen tension, and stay grounded.

1. Diaphragmatic Breathing

Begin via finding a quiet, snug region to sit down or lie down. Close your eyes and place one hand for your chest and the alternative on your belly. Take a sluggish, deep breath in through your nostril, allowing your stomach to rise as you fill your lungs. Exhale slowly via your mouth, feeling your stomach fall. Repeat this device, focusing on the upward push and fall of your stomach. With each breath, agree with liberating tension and strain.

2. Box Breathing

Box breathing is a method utilized by many to calm the worried device. It consists of a smooth 4depend sample.

Inhale for a recollect of 4.

Hold your breath for a depend range huge variety of 4.

Exhale for a remember of four.

Hold your breath for a depend of four.

Repeat this sample for numerous mins, steadily extending the length as you end up extra comfortable. Focus on your breath and the counting, allowing any racing thoughts to dissipate.

The Power of Mindfulness

Mindfulness is the workout of being actually gift in the 2d, watching your thoughts and sensations without judgment. It will let you reconnect together with your frame and launch anxiety.

3. Body Scan Meditation

Find a snug feature, both sitting or mendacity down. Close your eyes and produce your interest for your breath for some moments. Then, shift your popularity to your feet. Pay interest to any sensations or tension to your feet, and consciously lighten up them. Slowly artwork your manner up through every part of your body, releasing tension as you pass. This exercise enables you end up greater privy to physical sensations and promotes rest.

Body Scanning

Trauma frequently leaves a lingering imprint at the frame inside the shape of bodily sensations. Body scanning is a method that includes systematically checking in with particular factors of your body to recognize and release anxiety.

1. Progressive Muscle Relaxation

Begin with the useful resource of way of mendacity down or sitting in a snug characteristic. Close your eyes and take a few deep breaths. Start along side your feet and art work your manner up via your frame, tensing each muscle institution for a few seconds and then releasing. Pay close to hobby to the feeling of anxiety melting away as you allow bypass.

2. The Somatic Experiencing "Felt Sense"

Developed with the beneficial aid of Peter A. Levine, the "felt enjoy" is an exercise in which you find out your frame's sensations with out judgment. Close your eyes and attention on an area of your body that feels demanding or uncomfortable. Allow your attention to rest there, and try to word any diffused sensations or adjustments in that location. This exercise permits you connect with the frame's innate attention and might often display insights approximately underlying emotional anxiety.

Movement and Exercise

Movement is a effective device for reconnecting along side your body. When completed mindfully, it is able to release pentup feelings and repair a experience of safety and manipulate.

1. Yoga for Grounding

Yoga is a holistic exercising that mixes physical postures, breath manage, and meditation. It's specially effective for grounding as it encourages recognition of body sensations and breath.

Start with simple, grounding poses like Child's Pose, DownwardFacing Dog, or Warrior I.

Focus on your breath as you circulate via the ones postures, inhaling and exhaling deeply.

Imagine your self rooting into the earth with every posture, grounding your electricity.

2. Walking Meditation

Walking meditation is a mindfulness exercising that consists of on foot slowly and deliberately, paying whole hobby to every step.

Find a quiet direction or location to stroll.

Begin by using way of using taking some deep breaths, focusing your interest in your breath.

Start walking slowly, feeling each footstep connecting with the ground.

Notice the sensations on your feet and legs as they flow.

If your mind wanders, gently deliver your recognition returned on your taking walks.

Guided Visualization

Guided visualization is a technique that makes use of your imagination to create a feel of protection, consolation, and empowerment. By vividly imagining excellent research, you could reprogram your mind and frame's reaction to pressure and trauma.

1. The Safe Place Visualization

The Safe Place Visualization is a effective device to help you create a highbrow sanctuary wherein you could discover secure haven in times of misery.

Begin with the useful resource of locating a quiet, cushty area to sit down or lie down.

Close your eyes and take severa deep, calming breaths.

Imagine an area where you enjoy completely stable, constant, and at peace. This may be a actual place out of your past or an area in reality of your nonpublic introduction.

Picture the data of this region: the colours, textures, and sounds. Feel the warm temperature of the sun or the chill of the coloration.

Imagine your self absolutely found in this safe place, experiencing a profound sense of peace and rest.

Whenever you sense crushed or disconnected out of your frame, pass again to this solid location in your thoughts to reground yourself.

2. The Inner Healer Visualization

This visualization lets in you tap into your inner assets and set off your frame's natural restoration capabilities.

Begin with the useful useful resource of locating a cushty and quiet area to sit or lie down.

Close your eyes and take numerous deep, calming breaths.

Visualize a smart and compassionate decide interior your mind. This could be a mentor, a religious manual, or sincerely an picture that represents recuperation and attention.

Imagine this discern radiating recovery strength and love within the path of you. Feel their presence surrounding you with warmth and resource.

Allow yourself to gather this restoration energy, visualizing it moving into your body in which you want it maximum.

As you breathe deeply, recollect any bodily or emotional wounds restoration, and a sense of strength and peace spreading in the course of your frame.

Know that you may pass back to this internal healer visualization whenever you want help and recuperation.

three. Future Self Visualization

The Future Self Visualization is a device for putting intentions and envisioning your wonderful destiny.

Find a quiet and comfortable location to take a seat or lie down.

Close your eyes and take severa deep, calming breaths.

Imagine assembly your future self – a version of you who has healed and transformed beyond your present day struggles.

Engage in a verbal exchange along with your destiny self. Ask them questions about how they executed recovery and what steps you want to take to get there.

Feel the data and guidance of your future self as they provide insights and encouragement.

Visualize your self merging collectively together along with your destiny self, absorbing their strength, resilience, and optimism.

Carry this imaginative and prescient with you as a supply of motivation and concept in your recuperation adventure.

4. Releasing and Letting Go Visualization

This visualization enables you launch pentup feelings and negative strength from your frame.

Find a comfortable and quiet region to sit down or lie down.

Close your eyes and take numerous deep, calming breaths.

Imagine any emotional or physical tension on your frame as a cloud or a heavy weight.

Visualize this cloud or weight slowly dissipating or melting away, beginning from your ft and transferring up through your body.

As it dissolves, recall a sense of lightness and treatment changing the tension.

Continue this visualization until you sense a deep experience of relaxation and release.

Guided visualizations can be immensely powerful gadget for recovery trauma and reconnecting together together together with your body. The key's to exercise those bodily video video games frequently and tailor them on your unique dreams. As you hold your somatic remedy adventure, you can discover which visualizations art work superb for you and the way they may make a contribution for your emotional and physical restoration. In the following financial disaster, we are going to find out greater strategies to help you gather resilience and further beautify the mindbody connection.

Chapter 6: Building Resilience

Developing Resilience to Trauma

Trauma may be an excellent adversary, but it doesn't need to define your existence. Resilience is the important thing to no longer exceptional surviving however thriving after annoying testimonies. In this bankruptcy, we can discover strategies and practices that empower you to develop resilience, rebuild your life, and find out desire past the shadow of trauma.

SelfCare Practices

Selfcare is the cornerstone of healing from trauma and nurturing the thoughtsbody connection. It includes intentionally taking time to deal with your bodily, emotional, and psychological desires. While somatic therapy gives profitable equipment, selfcare practices can enhance and supplement your healing journey.

The Importance of SelfCare

Trauma often leaves people feeling depleted, emotionally tired, and disconnected from their our bodies. Selfcare practices are vital for rebuilding a sense of safety, keep in mind, and empowerment indoors oneself. They will can help you regain manipulate over your feelings and bodily sensations, permitting you to transport within the direction of recovery and increase.

Creating a Personalized SelfCare

Plan

1. Assessment and Reflection: Begin through assessing your present dayday selfcare conduct and their effectiveness. Reflect on what sports make you sense comfortable, grounded, and happy, and which ones can be triggers for strain or traumarelated responses.

2. Identify Your Needs: Everyone's selfcare desires are unique. Identify your unique dreams in the domains of physical, emotional, social, and spiritual nicelybeing. Consider what nurtures your thoughts, frame, and soul.

Physical SelfCare

3. Healthy Eating: Nourishing your body with balanced and nutritious food helps frequently happening nicelybeing. Pay attention to how sure components have an effect for your temper and power ranges.

4. Regular Exercise: Engaging in physical interest can release endorphins and reduce the bodily tension frequently associated with trauma. Find an exercise ordinary that fits your fitness stage and hobbies.

5. Adequate Sleep: Prioritize getting sufficient restorative sleep. Sleep is critical for emotional law and reminiscence consolidation, each of which might be laid low with trauma.

6. Mindful Movement:

Practices like yoga, Tai Chi, or Qigong permit you to reconnect together with your frame, release tension, and decorate flexibility.

Emotional SelfCare

7. Journaling: Keeping a magazine can offer a secure place to find out your feelings, track your improvement, and grow to be privy to patterns and triggers.

8. Creative Expression: Engaging in innovative sports consisting of paintings, music, or writing can be healing and help you unique emotions that can be difficult to verbalize.

9. Meditation and Mindfulness: Mindfulness practices will let you stay present, lessen tension, and control overwhelming feelings.

Social SelfCare

10. Boundaries: Establish and keep wholesome boundaries with others. Communicate your desires and boundaries honestly and assertively.

11. Support System: Build a network of supportive friends, circle of relatives contributors, or assist corporations. Connecting with others who've skilled trauma can offer a revel in of belonging.

12. Seek Professional Help: If essential, endure in mind treatment or counseling. A knowledgeable therapist can offer steerage and help tailormade to your particular stories.

Spiritual SelfCare

thirteen. Nature Connection: Spending time in nature can be deeply grounding and offer a revel in of peace and connection.

14. Mindful Practices: Engage in practices that align with your religious beliefs, whether it's far prayer, meditation, or mindfulness physical sports activities.

SelfCare as a Daily Ritual

Remember that selfcare isn't a luxurious; it is a want for recuperation. Create a each day or weekly selfcare routine that prioritizes your nicelybeing. Consistency is crucial to reestablishing a strong thoughtsbody connection and igniting the restoration method.

Key Takeaways

Selfcare is crucial for recovery from trauma and strengthening the thoughtsframe connection.

Assess your selfcare wishes and amplify a customised plan.

Address physical, emotional, social, and non secular nicelybeing in your selfcare regular.

Consistency in selfcare practices is crucial for lengthyterm restoration and growth.

Building a Support Network

In your adventure to heal from trauma the use of somatic therapy, one of the most crucial factors is putting in a robust useful resource community. While the strategies and sports activities you have were given positioned can be quite effective, the energy of a supportive community or network want to no longer be underestimated. Your manual network can embody friends, own family, assist corporations, or perhaps a therapist. Here, we discover the importance of this community and a manner to construct and nurture it.

The Importance of a Support Network

1. Emotional Resonance: A useful resource community gives a secure area an excellent manner to specific your emotions and research without judgment. Sharing your feelings with facts humans may be particularly therapeutic.

2. Validation: Trauma survivors regularly struggle with selfdoubt and emotions of isolation. Your help community can validate your opinions, supporting you comprehend which you are not on my own in your journey.

3. Stability and Consistency: Consistency is vital inside the restoration manner. A reliable manual network can provide stability on your life, supporting you sense more constant and levelheaded.

4. Accountability: Your help network can maintain you liable for yourselfcare practices and remedy durations, making sure you stay

heading inside the right direction along side your healing journey.

Identifying and Enlisting Support

1. Family and Friends: Assess your present day relationships and identify people who are honest and empathetic. Share your journey with the ones you revel in maximum snug with and who've a records of being supportive.

2. Support Groups: Support groups can be particularly beneficial for trauma survivors. These organizations consist of human beings who have had comparable opinions and might offer precious insights and empathy. Explore neighborhood and on line alternatives.

three. Therapists and Counselors: If you are operating with a therapist, they may be a crucial a part of your help community. Discuss the possibility of regarding a therapist in organization intervals or circle of relatives remedy to beautify information and assist from loved ones.

Nurturing Your Support Network

1. Effective Communication: Open and sincere conversation is the inspiration of a sturdy guide community. Express your wishes, limitations, and improvement to your help device.

2. Reciprocity: Remember that relationships are a manner avenue. Be inclined to offer help in move lower back and widely diagnosed the desires of your family as nicely.

three. Boundaries: Establish easy limitations inner your assist community. Make excellent you're snug with the quantity of involvement from every member, and speak those obstacles as wished.

four. Regular CheckIns: Maintain regular touch collectively together with your useful resource network. Whether through cellphone calls, conferences, or texts, staying associated allows build be given as true with and guarantees you have a dependable deliver of encouragement.

five. SelfCare Together: Consider conducting selfcare sports with individuals of your useful resource network. This can foster connection and create notable shared reviews.

When Support Network Falters

1. Addressing Conflicts: Conflicts can rise up even inner supportive networks. Learn battle decision techniques to keep the integrity of your network.

2. Seeking Professional Help: If your assist community isn't providing the important guide or turns into a supply of pressure, discuss together with your therapist for guidance on a manner to cope with the ones issues efficaciously.

Remember, constructing and retaining a assist community is an ongoing approach. It's a treasured useful resource in your recuperation journey, supplying comfort, understanding, and a enjoy of belonging as you find out the transformative electricity of somatic treatment.

Building Resilience

In our journey in the path of recuperation trauma and enhancing the thoughtsframe connection, one valuable beneficial aid we will draw upon is the field of splendid psychology. Positive psychology specializes in the strengths and attributes that permit people and groups to thrive, in preference to totally addressing troubles and issues. It gives a easy attitude on resilience, emphasizing no longer excellent bouncing over again from adversity however additionally growing and flourishing within the face of lifestyles's disturbing conditions.

The Power of Positive Psychology

Positive psychology is grounded inside the belief that humans have the ability for increase, change, and happiness, even within the wake of trauma and adversity. This phase explores how the ideas of excessive exceptional psychology may be covered into somatic remedy to enhance resilience:

1. StrengthBased Approaches

In conventional remedy, the focal point frequently centers on hasslesolving and addressing weaknesses. Positive psychology takes a totally precise course with the useful resource of emphasizing an individual's strengths, virtues, and skills.

Discover how identifying and nurturing your personal strengths can useful useful resource in resilienceconstructing. We'll discover carrying activities and strategies on the way to let you understand your specific traits and take a look at them to conquer demanding situations.

2. Positive Emotions and Wellbeing

Positive feelings play a vital role in building resilience. This a part of the economic spoil delves into the era of nice emotions, explaining how they impact our normal wellbeing.

We'll provide techniques for cultivating tremendous feelings, even inside the midst of trauma recovery. These strategies embody gratitude sports activities sports, savoring great experiences, and fostering a hopeful outlook at the future.

three. Mindset and Resilience

Your attitude can appreciably have an impact in your capability to bounce back from adversity. Positive psychology introduces standards like a boom thoughtsset and located updemanding increase.

Learn a way to shift your thoughtsset within the direction of boom and resilience. We'll provide sensible guidelines for growing a growth mindset and the usage of adversity as a catalyst for private improvement.

four. The Role of Positive Relationships

Social resource is a cornerstone of resilience. Positive psychology underscores the importance of nurturing healthy relationships and connections.

Discover a way to collect and preserve tremendous relationships that contribute for your resilience. We'll moreover discover the power of forgiveness and the way it could be a device for restoration and boom.

Integrating Positive Psychology with Somatic Therapy

Positive psychology is not a replacement for somatic therapy but instead a complementary approach. In this segment, we are able to guide you on integrating fantastic psychology standards into your somatic remedy exercise:

Creating a Positive Somatic Experience: Learn a manner to use somatic strategies to foster fine feelings and stories interior your frame. This includes combining mindfulness, frame reputation, and awesome affirmations.

Building a Resilience Toolbox: Develop a personal resilience toolbox that consists of every somatic sports activities and excellent psychology practices. This toolkit will empower you to navigate life's challenges with electricity and style.

Tracking Progress: Explore strategies for tracking your development in resiliencebuilding. Journaling and selfassessment machine will assist you study and feature amusing your increase.

By incorporating brilliant psychology into your somatic remedy adventure, you'll no longer handiest heal from trauma however moreover embark on a path towards more resilience and a more perfect lifestyles.

Positive Psychology and Resilience

Positive psychology is a subject of psychology that focuses on the observe of human strengths, properlybeing, and the elements that make contributions to a fulfilling existence. In the context of trauma healing and somatic remedy, highquality psychology plays a large role in building resilience and fostering emotional restoration. This monetary disaster explores the thoughts of wonderful psychology and the manner they may be performed to enhance the approach of restoration and private growth.

Understanding Positive Psychology

Positive psychology is a drastically contemporary branch of psychology that emerged within the overdue 20th century as a response to the conventional recognition on pathology and the remedy of intellectual infection. It seeks to understand the great components of human enjoy, such as happiness, wellbeing, strengths, and virtues. Here, we are able to delve into some key ideas:

1. Positive Emotions: Positive psychology emphasizes the importance of experiencing amazing feelings like joy, gratitude, and preference, as they make contributions to ordinary wellbeing.

2. Strengths and Virtues: Identifying and the use of one's personal strengths and virtues can bring about a greater enjoyable existence

and additional resilience in the face of adversity.

3. Optimism: A excessive pleasant outlook on lifestyles, characterized via optimism, can help people navigate hard situations with more ease.

Positive Psychology and Resilience

Positive psychology and resilience are carefully intertwined. Resilience is the potential to get better from adversity, adapt to tough conditions, and even make bigger more potent in the device. Positive psychology offers precious system and perspectives that may enhance resilience:

1. Cultivating Optimism: Learn a manner to foster a extra positive attitude, even in the face of trauma. Positive psychology techniques, collectively with reframing terrible thoughts and running inside the route of gratitude, can contribute to a more hopeful outlook.

2. Building Resilience thru Strengths: Identify your nonpublic strengths and virtues, and leverage them to triumph over limitations. We'll find out sports and strategies for spotting and the usage of your innate abilities.

3. Mindfulness and SelfCompassion: Mindfulness practices, a center trouble of highquality psychology, can help people become greater aware of their thoughts and feelings. Selfcompassion strategies teach us to deal with ourselves with kindness and records, that is important at a few diploma in the recuperation manner.

Practical Exercises and Techniques

This segment offers sensible carrying activities and strategies rooted in excessive nice psychology to foster resilience. Select a magazine or pocket ebook that you could use entirely on your exercising.

Practical Exercises and Techniques: Gratitude Journaling

Gratitude journaling is a clean however powerful exercising that could have a profound effect on your highbrow and emotional properlybeing. It entails often taking time to mirror on and write down the belongings you are thankful for to your life. This exercise can assist shift your awareness from negativity and pressure to positivity and appreciation. Here's a stepvia manner ofstep guide to get you commenced:

Step 1: Choose Your Journal

Select a magazine or pocket ebook that you will use absolutely on your gratitude workout. It can be a bodily mag or a virtual one, depending on your desire. The key's to have a committed place to your reflections.

Step 2: Set a Routine

Establish a normal normal on your gratitude journaling. It may be daily, weekly, or at any frequency that works for you. Consistency is greater vital than frequency, so pick out a time table you can stick with.

Step 3: Reflect and Write

When it's time to magazine, discover a quiet and snug location to sit down and mirror. Take a few deep breaths to middle your self.

Step 4: List Three to Five Things You're Grateful For

Write down 3 to five assets you are thankful for at that second. These can be massive or small, precise or stylish. The key's to consciousness on what truly brings you pride and appreciation. Here are a few prompts to help you get began:

What made you smile nowadays?

Who or what are you grateful for for your existence?

What clean pleasures introduced you happiness?

What stressful situations have you ever ever triumph over nowadays?

Step five: Be Specific and Detailed

As you write, try to be specific and sure on your descriptions. Instead of just saying, "I'm thankful for my own family," you could write, "I'm grateful for the nice and cozy hug my accomplice gave me this morning, making me sense cherished and supported."

Step 6: Reflect on Why You're Grateful

After listing each item, take a 2d to mirror on why you're grateful for it. What excellent impact has it needed to your lifestyles? How does it make you experience? This deepens your connection to gratitude.

Step 7: Express Your Feelings

Allow your self to definitely experience the gratitude as you write. Let the terrific feelings associated with the ones moments wash over you. This may be a deeply emotional and uplifting experience.

Step 8: Review and Repeat

Over time, observe your beyond entries. This can help you see styles of positivity for your existence and remind you of the matters you can have forgotten to realize. Don't hesitate to copy gratitude for the equal matters in the event that they keep to deliver you joy.

Tips for Success:

Don't determine your entries; there is no proper or incorrect way to exercising gratitude.

If you're having a tough day, attempt to discover even the tiniest topics to be thrilled approximately.

Share your gratitude exercising with a relied on friend or therapist to decorate its impact.

Use your gratitude mag as a deliver of idea and positivity, especially in some unspecified time in the future of tough instances.

Gratitude journaling may be a transformative exercise, assisting you shift your attention towards the exquisite components of your existence and selling emotional recovery. Over time, you could likely word expanded emotions of happiness and contentment as you come to be greater attuned to the blessings, irrespective of how small, that surround you.

Practical Exercise: Strengths Assessment

A Strengths Assessment is a effective device for spotting and knowhow your particular inclinations and attributes. By identifying and leveraging your strengths, you could enhance your resilience, increase selfself assurance, and make extra informed alternatives to your recuperation journey. This workout will manual you thru the approach of discovering your strengths:

Step 1: SelfReflection

Begin thru the use of finding a quiet, snug area where you may reflect in your existence memories. Take a few deep breaths to center your self and create a non violent, centered thoughtsset.

Step 2: Identify Strengths from Your Life

Think about moments in your existence on the identical time as you felt exceptionally assured, succesful, or pleased with your self. These may be associated with nonpublic achievements, art work, relationships, or some different problem of your existence. Consider the following questions:

When have I felt the most assured and empowered?

What are a few accomplishments I'm in particular proud of?

In what situations do I sense most like "myself"?

Write down precise times or research that come to mind. These may be large or small, current or from your past.

Step three: Identify Patterns

Review the tales you have got were given listed. Are there any commonplace subjects or styles? Do positive dispositions or skills generally seem for your moments of energy and self perception? These patterns regularly suggest your middle strengths.

Step four: Seek Feedback

Sometimes, others can provide precious insights into your strengths. Reach out to pals, family individuals, or colleagues and ask them for his or her mindset. What do they see as your strengths? Collect their feedback and examine it to your personal reflections.

Step 5: Use a Strengths Assessment Tool

Several mental checks and questionnaires are designed that will help you emerge as aware of your strengths. The VIA Survey of Character Strengths, created through top notch psychology researchers, is one such tool. You can locate it online and whole it to gain further insights into your strengths.

Step 6: Create Your Strengths Profile

Compile all the statistics you've got accrued about your strengths right right into a strengths profile. This may be a written file or a visible illustration, which includes a thoughts map or chart. Organize your strengths into classes if it permits you are making enjoy of them.

Step 7: Set Goals

Now which you have a clearer facts of your strengths, consider how you can use them to guide your recovery journey. Set specific goals that align in conjunction with your strengths, each in terms of personal growth and restoration from trauma.

Step 8: Apply Your Strengths

Incorporate your strengths into your each day lifestyles and healing practices. For instance:

If "empathy" is one in all your strengths, use it to deepen your connections along side your therapist and beneficial useful resource community.

If "creativity" is a electricity, explore innovative shops like artwork, track, or writing as a part of your recovery device.

If "resilience" is a center strength, consciousness on developing coping techniques that leverage this first rate in the course of hard moments.

Remember that your strengths can evolve and trade through the years. Continually revisit and replace your strengths profile as you make bigger and progress for your recuperation journey. Embracing your strengths may be a source of empowerment and motivation as you parent toward emotional and physical restoration.

Practical Exercises and Techniques: Mindfulness and Relaxation Practices

Mindfulness and rest practices are effective gear for decreasing pressure, growing selfattention, and selling emotional recovery inside the context of somatic remedy and trauma recovery. In this section, we are able to discover severa sporting sports activities and strategies that assist you to domesticate mindfulness and relaxation as a part of your recuperation journey.

1. Mindfulness Meditation

Mindfulness meditation is a foundational workout that includes paying centered hobby to the triumphing moment without judgment. This exercise may be particularly effective in calming the worrying device and lowering the effect of traumarelated strain. Here's a stepwith the useful resource ofstep guide:

Find a Quiet Space: Choose a quiet region wherein you won't be disturbed.

Get Comfortable: Sit or lie down in a snug feature. You can use a cushion or chair for resource.

Focus on Your Breath: Close your eyes and bring your interest on your breath. Notice the feeling of your breath because it enters and leaves your nostrils or the upward thrust and fall of your chest or belly.

Acknowledge Thoughts: When mind upward thrust up (and they will), famend them with out judgment and gently pass lower back your interest on your breath.

Body Scan: If you revel in snug, you could moreover do a frame experiment, wherein you systematically recognition your interest on each a part of your body, out of your feet for your head, noticing any sensations with out judgment.

Start Small: Begin with only some minutes a day and progressively increase the length as you turn out to be greater cushty with the workout.

2. Guided Relaxation Exercises

Guided rest bodily video video games are audio recordings or scripts that lead you thru a relaxation approach. These may be in particular beneficial even as coping with traumaassociated anxiety and tension. Here's the manner to apply them:

Find a Quiet Space: As with mindfulness meditation, pick out a quiet, comfortable place.

Select a Recording or Script: You can discover guided rest recordings on line or use a relaxation script. Ensure it's miles from an fantastic supply.

Follow the Instructions: Close your eyes, and listen or have a look at along because of the reality the guide takes you via a sequence of relaxation strategies. This can also include tensing and a laugh muscle businesses, deep respiration, and visualization.

Stay OpenMinded: Be open to the manner and permit your self to allow move of strain and tension.

Regular Practice: Consider incorporating guided rest into your every day or weekly normal for optimum gain.

Chapter 7: Integration And Self Healing

Integrating Somatic Therapy into Your Life

In the preceding chapters, we've got explored the profound functionality of somatic remedy to heal trauma and decorate the mindframe connection. Now, it is time to speak about how you could combine these powerful techniques into your day by day existence to acquire lasting transformation.

Daily Practices

Somatic remedy is simplest even because it becomes an important part of your every day recurring. Consider the subsequent practices:

Morning Rituals

Begin your day with grounding sports.

Practice mindfulness for the duration of morning exercises.

Mindful CheckIns

Regularly pause and song into your frame's sensations.

Acknowledge any developing feelings with out judgment.

Breath Awareness

Use conscious breathing techniques at some degree in the day.

Connect collectively along with your breath throughout moments of strain or anxiety.

Body Scanning

Conduct brief frame scans to discover tension or pain.

Release anxiety thru simple moves or stretches.

Journaling and SelfReflection

Journaling is a effective tool for selfdiscovery and healing:

Emotional Journaling

Write about your each day feelings and physical sensations.

Explore the connections among your emotions and bodily reviews.

Trauma Processing

Use journaling to way past stressful opinions.

Reflect on your development and insights over time.

Working with a Therapist

While selfpractices are treasured, operating with a professional somatic therapist can provide essential help:

Finding the Right Therapist

Seek a therapist with enjoy in somatic treatment.

Consider compatibility and be given as real with on your recovery courting.

Setting Goals

Collaborate at the side of your therapist to define your restoration goals.

Establish a remedy plan that consists of somatic strategies.

InPerson or Online Therapy

Explore the alternatives of inperson or virtual remedy.

Prioritize consistency and commitment in your remedy schooling.

The Ongoing Journey of Healing

Healing from trauma and nurturing your thoughtsframe connection is a lifelong adventure:

Patience and SelfCompassion

Understand that restoration takes time; be affected person with yourself.

Practice selfcompassion and selfforgiveness.

Embracing Growth

Embrace nonpublic boom as an ongoing manner.

Celebrate your milestones and successes, irrespective of how small.

Building Resilience

Continue to construct resilience thru selfcare.

Adjust your somatic practices as wanted over time.

Sharing Your Knowledge

Consider assisting others through sharing your somatic treatment stories.

Support others on their recovery trips.

Incorporating somatic remedy into your life is a transformative manner. It's about creating a conscious choice to prioritize your nicelybeing and harness the strength of your mindframe connection. Remember, restoration isn't always a vacation spot but a continuous evolution, and with determination and selfcompassion, you may revel in profound recuperation and private increase.

In the following bankruptcy, we are going to delve into reallifestyles case research and achievement testimonies to demonstrate the tangible impact of somatic treatment on people who've released into their own restoration trips.

Chapter 8: Case Studies And Success Stories

Real Life Transformations

In the adventure of recovery from trauma and enhancing the thoughtsframe connection via somatic remedy, it is frequently inspirational and reassuring to pay attention approximately actuallife fulfillment tales. In this bankruptcy, we delve into the recollections of people who've surpassed via profound adjustments the use of somatic treatment strategies. These case studies illustrate the power of the thoughtsbody connection and provide desire and steering to those on their recovery direction.

Case Study 1: Overcoming Childhood Trauma

Betty's Story:

Betty, a 38twelve monthsantique woman, had carried the heavy burden of youth trauma for optimum of her existence. She professional forget about and emotional abuse in some unspecified time in the future of her teens, leaving her with deep emotional scars. Traditional talk therapy had furnished some comfort, however Betty notwithstanding the fact that felt trapped in her past.

Through somatic therapy, Betty located out to reconnect along aspect her body and release the saved anxiety and feelings from her demanding past. Grounding carrying activities and mindfulness practices completed a pivotal function in her restoration journey. Betty's story highlights the significance of somatic remedy in addressing earlyexistence trauma and the lasting effect it may have on one's properlybeing.

Case Study 2: Healing from PTSD

Solomon's Story:

Solomon, a navy veteran, had served in a combat location, which induced him developing excessive signs and symptoms and signs of put upstressful pressure ailment (PTSD). His life grow to be Solomoned via flashbacks, nightmares, and a consistent nation of hypervigilance. Traditional therapy had supplied a few treatment, however Solomon end up searching out a greater holistic method to recovery.

Somatic treatment, with its attention on the mindbody connection, have become a exercisechanger for Solomon. Through strategies like body scanning and managed breathing, he located to adjust his hectic device's response to triggers. Over time, Solomon skilled a discount in his PTSD symptoms and symptoms and a newfound feel of control over his life.

Case Study 3: Thriving after Adverse Experiences

Lena's Story:

Lena, a survivor of a essential car coincidence, had skilled no longer only bodily trauma but moreover emotional scars from the incident. For years, she struggled with anxiety, melancholy, and chronic pain. Lena had attempted severa varieties of therapy and medication, but she but felt trapped in a cycle of suffering.

Somatic remedy introduced Lena to a wonderful way of drawing close to her recovery journey. She observed the profound connection amongst her emotional us of a and physical ache. Through somatic strategies and guided visualizations, Lena discovered to release the anxiety in her body and approach her feelings. Her story is a testomony to the transformative strength of somatic treatment in helping humans regain control over their lives after poor critiques.

Key Takeaways

These reallifestyles differences highlight the effectiveness of somatic treatment in addressing a extensive sort of traumas and worrying conditions. While all people's adventure is precise, the commonplace thread in those reminiscences is the profound effect of reconnecting with the frame, statistics the mindframe connection, and using somatic strategies to ignite restoration and transformation.

These case studies feature a reminder that recuperation is viable, even in the face of fantastic adversity. Somatic remedy gives a direction to now not highquality heal from trauma but also to thrive and lead a satisfying existence.

In the following financial ruin, we discover the idea of personal growth and transformation past recuperation, presenting insights and guidance for the ones searching out to encompass a brighter destiny.

Chapter 9: Personal Growth And Transformation

From Healing to Thriving

In the previous chapters, we have were given delved into the profound worldwide of somatic therapy and explored its applications in recovery trauma, fostering emotional nicelybeing, and enhancing the mindbody connection. Now, as we approach the culmination of this journey, we are able to shift our popularity from definitely recovery to actively thriving. This financial disaster will guide you thru the transformational way of now not best getting better from trauma however moreover transcending it, embracing nonpublic increase, and locating a route to a colorful and pleasing existence.

SelfDiscovery and Personal Growth

Embracing SelfDiscovery

In the pursuit of restoration, we frequently discover factors of ourselves that were previously hidden or suppressed. This newfound selfreputation is a effective tool for personal boom. We'll find out strategies and sports to keep this selfdiscovery journey, assisting you recognize your values, passions, and real self.

Setting Personal Growth Goals

Setting smooth and ability personal boom desires is important for transferring from restoration to thriving. We'll speak the way to outline giant desires and create a roadmap for sporting out them. Whether it is profession aspirations, contemporary endeavors, or nonpublic relationships, your goals may be your guiding mild.

Finding Meaning and Purpose

The Search for Meaning

Trauma can frequently go away us wondering the because of this of our reviews and the cause of our lives. We'll delve into existential questions and provide system to help you locate your unique experience of which means and purpose, even in the face of adversity.

Contributions and Giving Back

One of the most fascinating factors of thriving is contributing to the properlybeing of others. We'll explore the concept of giving decrease returned, whether or not or no longer or now not through volunteer work, mentoring, or sharing your tale, and the way it may supply a profound experience of reason and joy.

Embracing a Full and Vibrant Life

Cultivating Joy and Positivity

Thriving isn't pretty plenty surviving; it is about experiencing lifestyles to the fullest. We'll delve into techniques for cultivating pride, gratitude, and positivity in your each day life. By embracing those practices, you could decorate your trendy wellbeing.

Building Healthy Relationships

Healthy relationships are a cornerstone of a thriving existence. We'll communicate the importance of obstacles, effective communication, and selfcare inside relationships. Whether it's far with own family, friends, or a romantic accomplice, nurturing healthy connections is important.

Resilience within the Face of Challenges

Finally, we can discover how your newfound resilience can help you navigate destiny annoying situations with grace and power. You'll discover ways to adapt to lifestyles's united statesand downs, retaining your properlybeing even though confronted with adversity.

Resilience within the Face of Challenges

Resilience is the capability to bounce back from adversity, adapt to exchange, and preserve properlybeing inside the face of lifestyles's challenges. Building and nurturing resilience is a crucial trouble of transitioning from restoration to thriving. It equips you with the electricity to climate storms, increase from hard research, and maintain for your direction to a colorful existence.

Understanding Resilience

Resilience isn't always an inherent trait but a skill that can be superior and strengthened. It's now not approximately averting adversity; it's about the way you respond to it. Understanding the critical component components of resilience can help you domesticate it effectively:

1. Emotional Regulation

Learning to understand and control your feelings is fundamental to resilience. When faced with demanding situations, acknowledging your feelings and finding wholesome strategies to explicit them can save you emotional crush.

2. Adaptability

Life is unpredictable, and trade is regular. Resilient people are adaptable, able to modify their techniques and mindset even as times shift. We'll find out techniques for boosting your adaptability.

3. Social Support

Building and maintaining a assist network is crucial. We'll delve into the significance of trying to find help from pals, own family, or specialists on the same time as needed, and the way to foster the ones supportive relationships.

four. Problem Solving

Resilience includes effective troublesolving skills. You'll find out how to break down stressful conditions into viable steps and increase a proactive technique to overcoming boundaries.

5. Positive Outlook

Maintaining a top notch outlook, even in tough instances, can substantially impact your resilience. We'll talk strategies for cultivating optimism and wish.

Building Resilience

1. Mindfulness and Stress Reduction

Mindfulness practices, at the side of meditation and deep respiratory sporting sports, can assist lessen pressure and beautify emotional law. We'll offer stepby manner of way ofstep commands for incorporating mindfulness into your each day ordinary.

2. SelfCompassion

Being kind and compassionate to your self, specifically at the same time as going through adversity, is a key difficulty of resilience. You'll research techniques for education selfcompassion and selfcare.

3. Learning from Setbacks

Resilience isn't about avoiding failure; it is approximately studying and growing from it. We'll discover the manner to reframe setbacks as opportunities for personal development.

4. Developing Flexibility

Flexibility is critical for adapting to existence's curveballs. We'll communicate techniques for boosting your potential to alter your goals and plans whilst activities exchange.

5. Strengthening Social Connections

Your useful resource network performs a fullsize function in resilience. We'll offer steering on a way to nurture and boom your social connections, every in correct instances and for the duration of adversity.

Maintaining Resilience

1. SelfCare

Consistent selfcare practices are important for maintaining resilience. We'll discover numerous selfcare techniques, from exercising and nutrients to relaxation and interests.

Chapter 10: Somatic Mindfulness

The thoughts and the body are linked, and they'll be constantly speaking with every exclusive. People who battle to meditate because their minds are too active can advantage from a way that specializes within the body. It gives them some factor to pay interest on, this is beneficial. Instead of actively seeking to prevent your thoughts from racing, you may try bringing your interest once more for your frame and the way it's miles feeling in preference to actively looking to prevent your mind. When you are making room for physical hobby, you can come to the perception that you enjoy extra than you believe you studied you do, which might also assist you in experiencing a experience of stability, roundedness, and stillness.

Things do not usually circulate properly in lifestyles. It is not uncommon for us to lose tune of our bodies as we pass about our everyday lives. It's feasible that the matters that stress us out from the outdoor and the

106

things we need to do soak up extra of our highbrow power than how our worried gadget functions. When you exercising a form of meditation referred to as somatic, you calm your mind by first that specialize in thrilling your frame.

Somatic Experiencing

A form of complementary and possibility remedy known as somatic experience treatment is meant to facilitate the restoration machine for patients who have suffered some shape of trauma.

This remedy became superior through way of Peter Levine, who holds a PhD. It is based on the idea that worrying research depart an imprint on the body, which may be the idea reason of a number of the signs and symptoms that people who have PTSD or who've been via disturbing evaluations might also exhibit. People use this approach to paintings towards decreasing the outcomes of strain on their our bodies.

A splendid variety of humans who've been through stressful opinions, specially people who encompass bodily trauma which encompass sexual attack or domestic abuse, may additionally moreover grow to be alienated from their our bodies.

They are able to get a greater popularity of what is going on indoors of them (their interceptive, proprioceptive, and kinesthetic emotions) because of having somatic critiques.

Principles of Somatic Therapy

Your Body Speaks Through Sensation

They in no manner prevent complaining approximately how they may be feeling, whether it's that they are thirsty, hot, hungry, whole, heat, bloodless, thirsty, hurting, etc. There are moments whilst the message That hurts! Is quite clean. There are times at the same time as they are no longer efficaciously apparent.

And accept as true with it or no longer, your frame is able to talking masses greater than genuinely whether or not or now not it's far whole, thirsty, cold, warm, hurting, or hungry.

What does it revel in like?

A feeling that you have on your frame is called an emotion.

Sensation Language is a manner of speakme that uses phrases derived from the five senses (taste, contact, heady scent, sound, and sight) to deliver how certain physical sensations make you feel.

It is essential to preserve your emotions harm away how you feel approximately your self. Even even though we enjoy feelings alongside issue our feelings, our feelings themselves are not the identical element as our emotions.

Here are some more examples: The sensation of tingling is one. Anger is not. It makes one queasy. Longing is not. Be cushty with it. Happy is not.

In a nutshell, discussing Sensation includes drawing on language associated with every of the five senses so as to talk approximately the sensations that stand up inside the frame.

Your Body Speak Through Movement

The way we recognize our body can shift relying on the surroundings we're in or the sports we follow. Examines six "our our bodies" of knowledge that have an impact on how humans reflect onconsideration on our bodies.

These our bodies of know-how are the imagined frame, the purchaser body, the transgressive body, the managed frame, and the practiced body. The discursive frame is the 7th body of information.

The frame that is pictured is how a person imagines their very non-public frame seems to others from the outside, or how they take delivery of as genuine with one-of-a-kind humans view them.

This so-called frame is observed through the lens of the "panoptic gaze," it is a form of self-surveillance wherein a lady or lady observes her private body as despite the fact that thru the eyes of different human beings. Does she want to get a current cloth material cabinet? Do they make it appear like her legs are huge? This compassionate internal witness, which can be evolved through somatic practices consisting of Authentic Movement yoga or conscious psychotherapy, is a much cry from the internal gaze, which inspires human beings to take a look at their personal our our bodies with numerous tiers of distress for symptoms and signs of being terrific from an idealized image. This inner gaze encourages human beings to have a take a look at their private our our bodies with diverse levels of distress for signs and symptoms of being specific from an idealized photograph.

A "patron frame" is one which buys subjects or participates in sports activities sports activities (thru identifying with a group or through using going to a gym in the event that they see themselves as athletes) and sees their frame as an item that can be modified through exercise, food regimen, or surgical treatment to meet a nice "pleasant" goal. This definition applies to individuals who purchase topics or take part in sports sports (with the useful resource of identifying with a set or through going to a fitness center inside the occasion that they see themselves as athletes).

Some people don't forget that a frame that is managed and a frame that breaches the pointers are certainly two facets of the equal coin.

A frame this is going against what society considers to be proper and regular is called a deviant body. The frame that has been closely pierced and tattooed, the frame that has a disability, and the frame that has some of muscular tissues are all examples. On the opportunity hand, a "disciplined" body is one this is coerced into doing things like workout and looking what it consumes, or one which has been medicalized, or one in which the body is the goal and cause of strength, which incorporates a first-rate frame. These interpretations and connotations of accurate and horrible make me query in which someone's frame might probably wholesome within the occasion that they have been each "nicely" and "terrible." Take, for example, a disabled athlete who adheres to a regimented training software or food plan, or a dancer who has a hard and fast of tattoos and does the equal element.

A unique challenge rely is added up thru particular varieties of dancing as well. There is no doubt that dance belongs in the elegance of bodies which have been disciplined; in spite of the reality that, many dance practices have the functionality to purpose harm, and someone who engages in the ones practices might almost probable be walking outdoor of the societal norm; this can location them in the class of our our bodies that have transgressed social norms.

People have the false impression that a expert player has a "practiced frame" because of the truth they do things over and over till they turn out to be second nature.

Where obtaining the ideal social code of strength, self-self assurance, and region thru participation in a set is an important difficulty.

The social advantages of running in the direction of martial arts are frequently seen as having a better precedence amongst members than clearly enhancing one's bodily skills. This can be interpreted as a way in which physical hobby is applied as a social exercise to manipulate and have an effect on human beings and to get them to do what the ones in authority want them to do. In Tae Kwon Do, as in loads of diverse kinds of martial arts, there may be a splendid score tool. In addition to gymnastics and soccer, which can be every examples of different sports sports sports, there are different know-how development systems which may be organized in a hierarchy. How does this concept relate to other practices that call for professional movement and a "practiced body," but that don't manifestly adhere to this form of dogmatic stance?

This is similar to how Authentic Movement and distinct sorts of somatic expression use language to talk approximately what the frame evaluations. Because language plays this type of significant function in every our comprehension of and our enjoy of our our our bodies, we should in no way bargain its importance.

Body Boundaries

Establishing obstacles calls for first having a commercial enterprise organization keep close to on one's very non-public identification, in addition to one's personal necessities and desires, after which being able to articulate those necessities and goals. Every one mother and father has limits, and it is inevitable that we will have a number of those barriers tested finally.

People frequently have the faulty concept concerning obstacles. They receive as real with they have got wholesome boundaries, however in truth, they may be genuinely stone walls, or they consider rules to be unkind.

Setting suitable barriers is essential to the achievement of any relationship. Relationships do not feature nicely without smooth limits, that may bring about feelings of annoyance, dissatisfaction, or maybe of getting one's rights infringed. If you do not deal with the ones feelings, they may be able to make you experience reduce off from other people or entangled, that is on the equal time as your dreams and emotions integrate with those of various human beings. If you do no longer deal with the ones feelings, they're capable of make you sense reduce off from distinct people or entangled. Neither of these are brilliant positions to take.

Establishing barriers calls for first having a enterprise keep near on one's very very own identification, as well as one's personal necessities and dreams, after which being capable of articulate those necessities and desires. Every one humans has limits, and it's miles inevitable that we are going to have some of those limitations tested sooner or later.

The majority of the time, human beings do no longer intentionally breach your recommendations; instead, they achieve this because of the truth they will be blind to what they will be. Sometimes this takes region due to the fact we do no longer talk effectively with ourselves or others concerning the subjects that we need or require.

The following is a list of six limits that you are entitled to, along side an example of what each one might seem like in exercise.

Here Are Six Steps That Will Assist You in Establishing and Maintaining Healthy Boundaries

Physically delineated regions of territory

Your bodily limits consist of things like the requirements of your frame, along with the need to consume, drink, and get a few rest.

It is appropriate to allow others apprehend that you do not need to be touched or which you require more area from them. It is appropriate to unique that you are hungry or require a damage at any time.

The following are a few instances of healthful limits to at least one's physical interest:

I've been going nonstop for days. Please excuse me at the identical time as I pass discover a seat.

I am no longer a massive lover. I need to shake arms.

I'm hungry. I should get a few thing, so please excuse me.

Because I am allergic to pets, it isn't always steady for us to hold that in our house.

No. That isn't the way in which I need to be touched.

Do not input my room except I offer you with specific permission to reap this.

When a person violates your physical boundaries, it can feel like they'll be touching you in an unwelcome manner, telling you to maintain taking walks when you are tired or that you want to attend to eat or drink, or moving into your private place in a way that makes you enjoy uncomfortable, together with getting into your room with out your permission. The severity of this may range everywhere from mild to very extreme. The most severe forms of infractions may want to likely result in immoderate mistreatment or overlook of the body.

Establishing limits for one's emotions

The idea of emotional limitations refers back to the act of acknowledging, respecting, and honoring one's emotions and energy. Understanding how a splendid deal emotional strength you may control, knowledge while its proper to percentage and at the same time as it is no longer, and expertise how hundreds you can percentage with oldsters that don't respond properly are all a part of the process of setting emotional limits. When you respect the emotional limits of others, you validate their feelings and make sure you do not get inside the manner of their potential to soak up emotional information via now not interfering together with your personal.

It would possibly skip some thing like this:

When I inform you how I experience and you decide me, it motives me to completely shut down. I can extraordinary percentage this with you in case you take note of what I actually have to say and show right deference to me.

"I'm very sorry that you are going thru this type of hard time proper now. At this factor in time, I am now not prepared to absorb all of this information. Do you be given as proper with we're going to be capable of preserve discussing this at a later time?"

This is a hard time for me, and I want to talk plenty. Are you presently in a situation in which you are capable of pay hobby?

At this time, I am not capable to speak about that difficulty rely. This is not a pleasant time.

The following are a few examples of objects which could move beyond emotional limitations:

Sentiments being ignored and criticized in choice to mentioned

A failure to ask the quality inquiries concerning the relationship.

Going through information that is each non-public and emotional via studying or different approach.

Inquiring after people's sentiments through manner of inquiring how they enjoy

The illusion that we are able to recognize how one in all a kind human beings are feeling.

Communicating their thoughts and emotions to extraordinary human beings

Emotional dumping on different people without first acquiring their consent

You are supplying your kids with the wrong sort of emotional facts.

The constraints imposed with the aid of time

Because of the fee of it gradual, it's miles important that you workout warning in figuring out how you will spend it. The importance of enforcing time constraints cannot be overstated, whether or not at art work, at domestic, or with friends. When you vicinity remaining dates, it manner which you are aware of what factors of your lifestyles are most crucial to you and that you are ensuring that you have enough time to take care of all aspects of your existence without taking on too much. It is an entire lot much less complicated to speak to one-of-a-kind humans how an entire lot time you have to be had to spend with them even as you are aware about the topics which is probably maximum important to you.

The following are some instances of low-cost time constraints:

Unfortunately, I may not be able to make it to that occasion this weekend.

I can simplest live for the subsequent hour.

Would you be available for a verbal exchange in some time in recent times?

I'd perform a little element to be of assist, however if I did, I'd be asking too much of myself. Is there a possibility of a do-over?

Sundays are reserved for spending time with the own family, so we may not be able to make it.

I'll be pleased to help with that. "My fee in keeping with hour is...

When we violate time limits, we do such things as ask professionals for their time with out paying them, call for the time of different people, preserve people in conversations or on duties longer than we stated we would, show up overdue or cancel on human beings due to the fact we made too many plans.

In addition, we name humans after they have indicated that they may be busy.

The policies located on sexuality

There are a number of signs of real sexual barriers, including consent, settlement, and recognize, popularity of options and desires, and privateness.

The following are some examples of wholesome sexual limits:

Getting permission

Talking approximately the topics that make you glad and soliciting for the ones topics

You have the choice of asking for to use a condom in case you revel in the need.

Concerning the topic of birth control.

When you're announcing no to topics which you do no longer enjoy doing or that harm you, you are safeguarding the privateness of the alternative individual.

This may be interpreted as:

Are you interested by having sex at this very 2nd?

Are you thrilled with how this have become out?

Tell me about the subjects that you experience doing.

Tell me approximately what it's miles which you do not like.

I do not like that. Let's strive our hand at some difficulty else for a exchange.

I do not need to percentage a bed with you this night time, you stated. Instead, would you thoughts if we held fingers?

The following are some examples of crossing sexual obstacles:

You need to pout, chastise, or get indignant at the person in the occasion that they do not need to have sexual family individuals with you.

Lack of permission to do a little element

The coercion to engage in sexual sports which are in opposition to one's will

Unwanted sexual remarks or advances

Leering

A sample of mendacity approximately the usage of begin control

Providing faux records approximately your scientific statistics

Putting down or criticizing the sexual picks of some other individual

Without in advance consent, you couldn't contact, assault, or rape the sufferer.

The boundaries of human understanding

Your intellectual limitations are defined thru your thoughts, thoughts, and the extent of your hobby. Your healthful intellectual barriers might be broken when your thoughts and interest are neglected, driven down, or omitted altogether. Respect for the critiques of different people is an important problem of healthy intellectual limits. It is critical that there be mutual apprehend, similarly to a desire to engage in conversation and have a observe greater about one another.

A wholesome highbrow limit moreover requires one to do not forget whether or not or now not or no longer the present day moment is an appropriate one to speak about a particular trouble count number range.

It might be interpreted as:

I am conscious that you and I preserve remarkable critiques; however, I will now not will permit you to placed me down in this sort of manner.

I'd love to talk extra about this, however I do not count on thanksgiving dinner is the wonderful time to do so. I'd love to speak extra about this.

When we speak this subject count number, we do not make quite some headway. I do not recall that it is probably beneficial to talk approximately it currently.

I can recognize why we would come to big conclusions regarding this, you said.

Does this suggest that you need to be receptive to the hints and viewpoints of truely anyone? Absolutely now not even close to. Additionally, it is critical to collect the capacity to recognize the variations among wholesome and unhealthful verbal exchange.

You have each proper to attract a clean line within the sand if someone holds a negative opinion, at the side of racism, sexism, xenophobia, homophobia, or any of a number of other such perspectives. It is as much as you to choose how a long way you need to move. It must pop out as despite the fact that you are telling the person who you do now not experience that form of discourse, that you are pushing a long way from them, or that you are ceasing to speak to them. It isn't critical so that you can interact in highbrow speak with individuals who motive you or others damage.

Boundaries composed of physical gadgets

Material constraints embody subjects that you non-public together with your property, vehicle, garments, rings, fixtures, cash, and unique possessions. It is useful to have a smooth know-how of what can be shared and what can't, similarly to the way in that you would love the others with whom you percentage your home to deal with them.

Putting regulations at the techniques in which your belongings may be applied is beneficial and stops you from becoming indignant over time.

This is probably interpreted as:

I am now not able to lend my car to anyone. I am the exceptional one who is protected with the resource of the insurance.

We are out of coins and no longer able to offer any more. We is probably glad to assist in some other way that we are capable of.

Sure! It is probably my pleasure to lend you my dress. To let you understand that I do need it once more by way of Friday, that is only a heads up.

Your fabric limitations are being exceeded each time your property are broken, stolen, or borrowed on an overly common foundation. It is also a very extreme rely to use fabric gadgets, which consist of cash and possessions, to govern and control interpersonal connections.

When we installation barriers, we sharpen our attention of these limits, we not best make it a lot less difficult for one among a kind humans to be there for us, but we additionally enhance our functionality to be there for extraordinary people.

Trust Your Body's Impulses

Impulsivity is the tendency to act with out first thinking subjects through, which encompass whilst a person blurts out a few issue, makes an unplanned purchase, or runs all through the road with out looking both methods.

This sort of behavior, particularly at the equal time as it comes from children or young adults, isn't generally an instance that there is probably problem. They are liable to impulsive conduct due to the reality that their brains are though growing. However, in some times, it may be a symptom of a particular illness. When human beings do not assume in advance than they act.

People are infamous for making statements or taking moves that they later come to regret. However, there are some folks who engage in volatile conduct on a regular foundation, even on a every day basis. This form of conduct may additionally get you into problems and make you sense terrible about your self.

It is feasible that there can be an problem if any of the subsequent matters get up often:

Aggressive behavior

Agitation that motives troubles for precise humans

Being susceptible to a loss of interest

Situations that might motive a person to act in an impetuous way

There are an entire lot of fitness situations that may be indicated by way of impulsive behavior. In addition, it can get up itself in those who struggle with tension, autistic spectrum sicknesses, or substance abuse. The following are some of the maximum not unusual:

Attention Deficit Hyperactivity Disorder

It is cited via its acronym, ADHD. Interrupting precise humans on the identical time as they are speakme, shouting out answers to questions, and having issues geared up your turn in line are all symptoms of being impulsive. Interrupting other human beings while they may be talking approximately themselves is also an instance.

Bipolar infection.

This neurological circumstance alters the way you revel in, the amount of strength you've got were given had been given, and the way properly you could carry out the obligations of each day life. An example of impulsive behavior would be spending hundreds of cash on vain objects or making use of unlawful tablets.

Behavior troubles which can be antisocial in nature.

If you have were given the shape of conditions, you each don't care about doing the proper problem in any other case you do not care the least bit. You additionally will be predisposed to act poorly in the direction of various human beings without giving any belief to the capability consequences of your moves. They also can have interaction in risky behaviors such as drug usage or unique possibly dangerous sports at the spur of the immediately, and they will additionally warfare to maintain healthy private relationships.

Problems in being capable of control one's impulses

The frequency of those troubles has drastically decreased. People who've them have the enjoy of being compelled to act in tactics which might be dangerous to themselves or to others, that aren't socially nice, or which is probably a criminal offense. They can tackle some of appearances, which consist of the subsequent examples:

Intermittent explosive contamination.

This refers to a propensity to experience anger often, albeit it usually most effective lasts for brief periods of time. Even insignificant stimuli have the ability to set it off.

Trichotillomania.

This scenario, moreover known as "hair-pulling disease," takes area at the equal time as a person cannot manipulate the urge to take out hair from any a part of their frame, together with their head, eyebrows, eyelids, or special regions in their body.

Kleptomania.

When this takes area, you may not be capable of manage the need to scouse borrow, however whilst you do it, you will enjoy a experience of relief regardless of the truth that you won't be able to hold what you take.

Pyromania.

This refers to a desire to create fires or an obsession with doing so in a unmarried's lifestyles. It does no longer appear very frequently. Only approximately three percentage of sufferers admitted to highbrow hospitals are given a analysis of pyromania.

I can't save you gaming.

Persons will now and again make little bets on handshakes or play the occasional office pool, but people with this circumstance can get so stuck up in it that it affects their paintings or relationships and makes them sick from the strain. People will frequently make modest bets on handshakes.

Being organized for situations that require you to take fast movement is some other useful method. For example, you can supply a notepad with you and use it to doodle in it as a way to bypass the time. Alternatively, you may write some aspect down in advance than you assert it aloud.

The purpose of pausing for a quick time frame earlier than reacting rashly is to offer oneself the possibility to mirror on whether or not or no longer the motion they are approximately to take is a superb concept and to do not forget the ability results of such an movement.

How Your Body Stores Information

When you pass by your antique immoderate college, recollections of the chronic bullying, the person who wouldn't acquire "no" for a solution, and the immediate even as your instructor introduced to the complete class that you failed your very last exam come to mind.

You are experiencing knots in your stomach and feature the sensation that you are approximately to bypass out. The agonizing reviews you have got had and the anxiety they have got brought approximately do not virtually live for your mind. They are also preserved inside the frame within the form of reminiscences.

How Memories Are Recreated in Flashbacks

A flashback is what takes vicinity to us while some component from our records brings up ugly memories of the past. People, places, and topics that deliver up recollections from the beyond are generally called "triggers," and that they have got the functionality to motive a response in every our bodies and our minds.

It's feasible that we do not apprehend how the purpose ends within the response, however it's also possible that we do. Things that do not have whatever to do with what we went through however make us consider it can cause reminiscences of that experience, which can be known as flashbacks. It's additionally viable to have a flashback without being prompted through something in the outdoor worldwide or because of unwelcome thoughts.

The intensity of a flashback may be so severe that it nearly makes you experience as if you are reliving the worrying enjoy all all over again. The majority of the time, flashbacks are added on by means of using reminiscences of disturbing testimonies, and that they entail seeing tremendous gadgets. If you have got ever been worried in an car twist of fate, you may experience emotions of tension and anxiety on every occasion you're in a moving car. You may honestly have clean memories of what befell, almost as in case you have been experiencing it all once more. And at the same time as this happens, your body can also additionally additionally behave the same way it did even as it come to be going thru the painful experience.

Our minds and our bodies will be predisposed to get stressed approximately the time of day and whether or not or no longer some aspect is clearly taking region. It is viable for us to have the impact that we're reliving previously distressing critiques. The fact that the entire body is reacting on this way is evidence of a somatic memory.

Recollections of Past Emotions

People who have been via multiple worrying evaluations, specifically in the event that they commenced out when they had been greater younger, have an accelerated hazard of developing a shape of put up-traumatic pressure contamination known as C-PTSD, which stands for complicated PTSD. C-PTSD can regulate how a person feels approximately themselves and the world round them. People who suffer from complex positioned up-stressful strain ailment (C-PTSD) can also experience very effective flashbacks that don't usually comprise snap shots but though depart them feeling very dissatisfied or indignant.

A powerful emotional response that might linger for a great quantity of time can be prompted with the useful useful resource of reminders of earlier trauma. In addition, there isn't always typically an obvious connection a number of the stimulus and the response, which makes it extra tough to exert manage. It's possible which you have been made aware about a few aspect out of your beyond, and as a stop result, you skilled pretty a few wrath, worry, and disgrace. You won't have recalled (or done again in your thoughts) a specific occasion, but your body senses hazard, and your emotions shift as a result. Dealing with emotional flashbacks may be hard considering there isn't always an obvious connection between what brings decrease back the sensation and the way severe it's miles. This could make it tough to recognise a way to answer to the experience at the same time as it resurfaces.

Your Body Has Inborn Ways for Healing

Watch what you're wondering.

Your mind might also want to have an effect on the manner your frame features. When you observed indignant, impatient, or frustrated thoughts, your frame responds via way of way of liberating hormones collectively with adrenaline, cortisol, and norepinephrine, all of which is probably detrimental on your fitness. The manufacturing of experience-real chemical compounds like endorphins via way of your brain in reaction to effective questioning is related to advanced physical and mental health.

Establish a sincere technique to address fear and clear your thoughts of bad mind, collectively with engaging in every day exercising or meditating on immoderate best affirmations. Even if you simplest provide your self five mins to meditate each day, this could be like taking a "highbrow bathe" that washes away all the poisonous and negative thoughts which have collected to your mind at some point of the day.

Chapter 11: Somatic Breath Art Work

Sensory Motor Amnesia

Sensory-Motor Amnesia (SMA) takes place at the equal time as applicable fearful device rhythms come to be so conversant in each distinct that they cannot be adjusted on their private. More especially, the relationship between the neurological system and the somatic muscle machine loses control.

SMA Function

Muscles cannot decide what to do until a message from the mind is sent via the concerned tool. Nerves adventure to muscular tissues and pass returned to send and get preserve of messages from them. This is how we apprehend our personal our our our bodies. We can come across if a muscle is tight or free due to the truth we've got were given an internal feeling referred to as "soma" or "proprioception." As we improvement thru lifestyles, we studies new hobbies and responsibilities. Our brains recollect those responsibilities so we do now not want to relearn them on every occasion we want to carry out them. This is usually a first-rate trouble, however every so often we draw near right away to lousy behaviors.

When we repeat the same hobby in our each day life, or while we react rapid to an twist of destiny or to protect ourselves from an damage, our brains may additionally come to be "caught" in that behavior, setting the routine sample into our unconscious and out of our control.

Even while the muscle groups now not want to agreement, the mind keeps to inform them to. This disrupts the neurological device's remarks loop, inflicting the brain to overlook that the muscle is tightened. The thoughts believes that the muscle is snug, and no quantity of rub down or relax will alternate it. Pandiculation can be beneficial in this case.

CSE and Pandiculation can beneficial useful resource within the treatment of SMA inside the following strategies:

1.   Pandiculation lets in the mind and muscle tissues to talk with every other. It is a part of our proprioception, or first-man or woman popularity of ourselves. From a 3rd-character attitude, in case you sincerely said "loosen up" in your muscle groups, the muscle would likely not be capable of pay attention or apprehend what you stated. To regain manage of our muscle tissues, we need to use proprioception. We can reactivate the neural device by means of way of contracting the SMA-affected muscular tissues deeper into their everyday sample. The mind can restore control of the muscle twitch. The mind continues the enter loop to and from the muscle and resets the extent of what it acknowledges as a "comfortable" and a "contracted" muscle by using manner of frequently freeing the muscle from that deep contraction. This is referred to as a pink herring.

2.   Daily somatic bodily games and explorations assist to set up those healthful rhythms and avoid SMA. It is right to workout

first issue in the morning. When we sleep, our brains "turn off" our voluntary concerned device, preventing us from transferring our muscle companies. When we wake up inside the morning, we skip again to "on line," which means that every one of our behavior are right away to be had to be used. When we undertake Somatic Explorations first hassle inside the morning, our brains studies this. We assume that via schooling the mind useful conduct at this "boot up" second in the morning, we can be able to save you SMA from growing detrimental behavior.

Somatic Pandiculation

Pandiculation is what animals like cats and dogs do when they relaxation. They are NOT stretching; they may be pandiculating. They tighten and unfasten their back and front muscle tissues, which wakes up their nerve structures. We do a whole-frame yawn within the morning. First, we tighten our muscle organizations, then we stretch them, and then we absolutely loosen up.

In Somatics, we use this pandiculation approach to move thru the 3 predominant reflex patterns, retraining the thoughts to retrain our muscle groups to really lighten up and enlarge once more. When you provide your complete interest to what you're doing, you may permit pass of the concerns of regular lifestyles. This offers you a top notch destroy and a experience of rest.

Which 3 are the maximum vital?

Reflex Red Light

The muscular tissues at the the the front of the frame tighten no longer most effective as a startle response to fear, anxiety, and emotional upset, however also as a muscle version to an excessive amount of computer and cell cellular cellphone use. This slumped ahead posture can reason persistent neck, shoulder, and decrease once more ache due to the fact the shoulders spherical ahead, the pinnacle pokes forward, and the chest vicinity is compressed. It can also make it difficult to respire absolutely. Breathing too shallowly can maintain the frame from getting the air it needs to artwork nicely.

Reflex Green Light

When we bypass forward, the muscular tissues inside the decrease back of the frame tighten. When we walk, run, arise right away (suppose navy stance), or sit up, we are able to overcontract our again muscle agencies. If we attempt this often, it can bring about lower once more, neck, and shoulder pain, issues with our discs, and ache in our sciatic nerve. When we've got were given those forms of pains, it may be smooth to get depressed, demanding, or have problem dozing. Pain can begin to repeat itself.

Trauma reflex

It is the body's way of averting ache. When an coincidence or damage takes location, muscle companies on the edges of the frame tighten to avoid ache even more. Also, normal stresses like sporting a little one on one hip or having a challenge where you use one side of your body greater than the other can motive muscle organizations on that facet of the frame to tighten and rise up. Sports like tennis, golf, or swimming, gambling an tool like the guitar, or doing some factor else in that you might in all likelihood turn to one problem more than the other, can purpose a sprained ankle. All of those repeated moves and positions can purpose ache and make it hard to transport around inside the frame.

Chapter 12: Ptsd And Attachment Trauma
The Fight, Flight, Freeze or Fawn Response

The autonomic annoying tool controls physical features which include respiration, pulse price, perspiration, urine manufacturing, and digestion. This gadget operates invisibly to keep you transferring. When a stimulus overpowers this device, the sympathetic nervous device assumes control. This autonomic reaction controls the somatic responses of the body.

Several physical adjustments can upward push up even as the sympathetic fearful tool is lively: your pulse rate will boom, your adrenaline starts offevolved pumping, you shake and sway, you sweat more and breathe quicker, and your body famous a manner to deal with the stress. As a manner of self-safety, it employs a trauma reaction or a mixture of trauma responses. When the perceived hazard has passed or faded, the parasympathetic worried machine takes over to move again you to a normal state.

People discover ways to behave in this manner. A man or woman's upbringing, surroundings, way of life, and existence reports all play a characteristic in triggering a trauma reaction.

As a little one develops, they require compassionate care. The way wherein mother and father nurture their youngsters and manage social problems has a giant effect on their emotional intelligence. Your thoughts's amygdala is responsible for rational cognition. When intense emotions take control, you revert to the responses which have stored you strong inside the beyond.

Activating the Fight Response

The fight response is a self-shielding reaction to trauma wherein the man or woman acts aggressively toward the peril which will maintain safety. Increased cortisol and adrenaline levels make it more difficult to suppose certainly and act lightly. You specific your wrath through dominance and a desire for control. This is a possible fight reaction:

Impulsiveness and hypersensitivity, along with repelling someone the instant they touch you.

Using your frame to defend in opposition to a threat through watching at someone or speakme sharply.

Saying "No!" to a person who might not go away you on my own

Refuting an accusation which you were answerable for some thing.

Attempting to reveal your characteristic or continuing an trouble after it has ended.

Taking the initiative and coaching others what to do Self-sabotage: selecting conflicts with others over trivial or fabricated topics

Even despite the fact that combating also can seem like an beside the point response, there may be no longer some issue wrong with adopting a protecting posture. This is extensively proper during combat and wonderful existence-threatening situations.

But shouting, starting up fights, and announcing hurtful matters aren't powerful techniques of communication.

If you find out it difficult to overcome or avoid the fight response, strive:

Close your eyes, take deep breaths, and shipping your mind to a happy region.

Count to ten earlier than you communicate; in case you're however livid, do not forget to one hundred.

Using physical interest, including taking walks or dancing, to self-regulate and express emotions.

How the flight reflex function

The flight response is a trauma reaction dominated with the aid of way of avoidant, frantic behavior. It makes you need to run an extended way from the perceived danger. When provoked, it could be difficult to sit down down nevertheless, stay but, or maybe communicate with others. Restlessness, darting scholars, and trembling fingers and legs are all bodily manifestations of the stress response. This response may additionally moreover even result in chronic ache. The response to flight can resemble:

They try and keep away from perceived risks, including loud sounds in public.

Attempting to avoid condemnation with the resource of being best

Obtaining a manner to hold your thoughts off subjects

In a eating place or extraordinary congested setting, it's far prudent to stand the go out.

It is hard to conceive of something apart from the trigger

Trouble resting, exciting, and getting a few rest

Enhanced vigilance and agitation

Thoughts which can be racing or excessive.

Attempting to assuage anxiety with tablets or alcohol.

In situations alongside facet natural screw ups or threats to public safety, the flight response is suitable. But being by myself and heading off human beings can harm relationships, manifesting as stonewalling and making it hard to talk with others. If you locate it tough to conquer or keep away from the combat response, strive:

Self-assure that you are secure

Utilizing grounding strategies consisting of earthing, forest breathing, and rain remedy

You can lessen your prolonged degrees of anxiety via yoga or meditation.

How the Freeze Reaction paintings

The freeze response is a trauma reaction that makes use of dissociation to guard the person from an coming close to near danger. The flight reaction yields to immoderate task, while the freeze reaction rejects it with the useful resource of rendering you impassive and setting apart you from truth. People often are searching for advice from this as a "deer in headlights," and some say it resembles an animal that acts useless even as being pursued with the aid of an aggressor. You revel in immobilized and now not able to escape the peril. Your heartbeat will boom, your respiration hastens, and you sense as although you aren't to your private frame.

Here is an example of the halt response:

Having problem expressing feelings, together with talking in a monotone.

Selective mutism or now not talking finally of times of duress

You emerge as weary of making choices because it turns into extra tough to choose.

Brain fog is ambiguity, forgetfulness, and problem focusing.

Not being precise in discussions

Despair and falling asleep

Having hassle making or preserving plans

Times without a tremendous activities

Daydreaming constantly

Not taking over the telephone and failing to talk what you require

Attempting to escape fact via excessive use of narcotics, alcohol, video video video games, or television

For a person who perceives others as risks, the freeze response also can feel herbal and solid. However, it regularly outcomes in passivity in relationships which can be toxic.

Focus on self-recognition and take note to govern a freeze response with out setting apart your self or fleeing your issues.

Grounding Exercise

When human beings are irritating, they regularly lose touch with the on the spot and begin thinking about terrible reminiscences or issues approximately the future. Grounding exercise workouts are supposed to convey you decrease lower back to the present 2d and assist you cope with stress and anxiety.

Grounding physical activities are highbrow and physical obligations that help humans cope with strain and tension. Grounding carrying sports are frequently advocated by means of using manner of highbrow and behavioral fitness professionals for humans with hundreds of pressure and tension, particularly the ones who have been via trauma.

When your thoughts is whole of traumatic thoughts, grounding can bring you lower back to the present and make you experience more on pinnacle of factors of your frame.

Grounding responsibilities are intended to help you prevent considering lousy or stressful topics thru way of creating you greater privy to your surroundings. Some techniques to do which are to take deep, timed breaths and attention on how your toes sense on the ground.

These responsibilities can help humans with a big variety of intellectual health problems, collectively with PTSD, tension, despair, and addiction. It can also assist human beings with dissociative sickness, a scenario in which human beings lose contact with their thoughts, feelings, and sense of self.

Grounding movements can assist with bodily troubles like chronic pain and nausea because of chemotherapy through giving the frame a preferred damage.

Chapter 13: Techniques To Get Better And Heal From Trauma

Qigong and Shaking Practice

The body shaking exercise is the best and maximum all-encompassing shape of Qigong. Your body will gain the advantages of this in a large number of processes, and it'll additionally help cast off power blockages.

One of the number one benefits that comes from doing this exercise is stepped forward stages of relaxation.

Effortless and Uncomplicated movement

The truth that it's far both clean and herbal, which means that that earlier understanding isn't always important, is the single maximum vital detail. There is neither a concept nor a technique; there isn't always some element.

In factor of truth, in case you had been a mean, wholesome toddler who grew up and finished out of doors, you will likely have finished so on motive no matter the fact that you had been no longer even conscious which you had been doing it.

Aside from that, it's far thrilling, and if crucial, it can assist to result in a revel in of calm. When we have been younger, I'm relating to the years amongst early life and puberty, and every now and then even earlier than the age of 7, we used to interact in a number of "Qigong" sports, all of which regarded quite normal on the time.

Somatic Yoga

The fields of bodywork, motion remedy, and speak remedy are all added together beneath the umbrella of the take a look at and exercise known as somatic.

It encourages you to be privy to and act upon the emotions that stand up inner you. "Body" is translated from the Greek word "soma." Through the exercise of somatic, you becomes aware about your physical, intellectual, and emotional comfort zones, and thru the exercise of mindfulness, you may study wherein and the way you hold strain, trauma, and pleasure to your body.

This may be step one closer to letting skip of vintage recollections and patterns, bringing your body and thoughts into stability, entering into contact with the feelings and instincts on your intestine, and, in the end, feeling greater effective and complete.

In the Nineteen Seventies, Thomas Hanna, a researcher and lecturer within the Western international, modified into the primary character to location down the pointers for the movement device and the philosophy of somatic.

He advanced the method simply so the mind-body link, movement, and speak to may additionally facilitate the frame's natural restoration process and decrease the feeling of ache.

Movement Base Techniques

Squat

The first kind of motion is the lunge. During a squat, the hips and knees bend, which lowers the body's middle of gravity. Most of the paintings within the squat is done with the aid of the quads, hamstrings, glutes, adductors, and belly muscle corporations.

Training with squats makes it much less tough to rise up from a sitting position.

Squat Exercises:

Goblet Squat

Box Squat

Landmine Goblet Squat

Bend

Bending is the second one motion of the lower body. It consists of bending your hips at the equal time as preserving your knees although, and it simply works your glutes, legs, and middle. The maximum famous workout for bending is the deadlift.

Every day, you operate the bending movement whenever you pick out something up off the ground.

Bend Exercises:

Good Morning Russian

Kettlebell Swing Hip

Thrust Bent Knee

Lunge

It is the very last motion pattern for the decrease frame. It's a manual habitual for the squat and bend, so that you need to use your middle and legs to hold your self solid.

In everyday life, the stretch is used to climb stairs or a mountain.

Lunge Exercises:

Step-up Kettlebell

Split Squat Front

Rack Split Squat

Core

The fourth sample is involvement at the maximum easy degree. The torso, that's the location the various fingers and the legs, is crafted from a complex group of muscle corporations called the middle. Its important mission is to keep the spine stable in both although and shifting positions.

You do most of your every day things that involve the middle. It's the number one way to keep subjects constant and lets in deliver huge loads at the same time as doing out of doors art work or moving.

Core Exercises

Side Plank

Front Plank

Farmers Shoulder

Push

The thrust is the primary rhythm for moving the better frame. It is any motion in which you float a load or your personal frame weight faraway from you. When you push, you determine your fingers, shoulders, and center.

In regular lifestyles, the thrust occurs even as you open a door or rise up from mendacity for your again.

Push Exercises

Bench Press Squat

Dumbbell Press

Landmine Press

Pull

The very last aspect the better body does is pull. It is any motion in which you pull a load or your very own frame weight in the direction of you. Pulling actions paintings the biceps and the better lower again.

When a trash bag is taken out of a trash can, it is usually finished in the identical way.

Pull Exercises

Pull-up Bent-Over

Barbell Row

Sitting Band Row

Cyclical

This movement happens in cycles and is used to get from one area to each unique, like at the same time as you walk or run.

Your motion can be better for the rest of your lifestyles if you workout this sample.

Locomotion Exercises

Airbike Rowing

Biking trauma

Clearing shaking

Somatic Art Therapy

Somatic treatment, which have become developed by using Dr. Peter Levine and is likewise called "somatic experiencing," employs the thoughts, body, and spirit to useful useful resource in the recovery of people.

Reuniting the thoughts and frame calls for a body-centered method on the way to deal with various highbrow health issues.

In an entire lot of techniques, somatic remedy can useful resource humans handling pressure and highbrow fitness troubles.

Benefits of somatic remedy

1. Be aware of your body structure

Somatic treatment is a technique for developing body and mind focus. Traditional talk remedy can assist humans overcome highbrow and emotional problems, but somatic remedy can assist with worrying recollections held in the nervous tool.

Somatic treatment strategies:

This method allows human beings stay grounded inside the present.

Grounding

It is useful for humans with anxiety or flashbacks as it makes use of physical sensations to calm those emotions. Some techniques encompass strolling water over the hands and tensing and interesting diverse body elements. This redirects your interest to the present sensations and gets rid of your thoughts from past events.

Capitalization and useful useful resource allocation

When you're experiencing frightening thoughts or emotions, visualisation and resource control allow you to revel in stable and calm. You can accomplish this with the aid of manner of visualizing yourself in definitely glad instances, locations, or with satisfied humans.

Body exams

A body take a look at lets in you to assess your frame and decide wherein you experience ache or deliver tension. Find a comfortable function, whether or now not or not seated or mendacity down, and attention for your body from the feet up. This undertaking want to take in to thirty minutes due to the truth you ought to now not hurry. Take word of every physical and highbrow sensation you enjoy, even though it hurts or makes you enjoy uneasy.

2. Adapt and overcome trauma

Somatic remedy has been demonstrated to assist human beings with PTSD cope with their symptoms and signs and symptoms and allows many humans reconnect with their our bodies. This may be difficult for the ones who have suffered bodily harm, along side via domestic or sexual violence.

Somatic treatment operates on the idea that trauma is retained in the frame and dreams to modify this dysregulation. It makes you privy to how your body reacts to pressure and stimuli and demonstrates how your thoughts and movements can adjust this reaction.

Somatic therapy can assist people in overcoming trauma via making them privy to in which it is contained in their our bodies. This may be finished through mindfulness or meditative moves, in conjunction with yoga or tai chi.

3. Provide yourself with the sources you need to decorate.

Trauma can prevent us from living complete, satisfied lives to the fullest quantity possible. But somatic treatment can provide us with the equipment vital to beautify our mental fitness and eliminate the intellectual, emotional, and bodily barriers that prevent us from doing so.

Even although somatic experiencing informs us of tactics our our our bodies sense and the vicinity of our primal emotions, it moreover equips us with the way to control and method the ones emotions. Numerous somatic strategies, in conjunction with grounding and resourcing, can be accomplished at home or at the administrative center, allowing you to apply them every time you want to lighten up after experiencing a motive.

four. Release Stress

Somatic experiencing is one method to help the body in liberating the stress because of trauma. Mindful somatic sports can help with this because they heighten frame recognition and make it simpler to find out tight or sore areas.

People who've expert strain within the beyond can also furthermore have problem regulating their feelings, that would purpose bodily tension.

This includes the pause reaction, an opportunity to combat or flight. If a person feels threatened, they pause in place of combat or flee. The mind is incapable of spotting that someone isn't in chance. Therefore, the freeze response keeps, resulting in signs and symptoms and signs and symptoms and signs and symptoms together with disorientation, disconnection, and problem moving.

Experiencing somatically is an powerful approach for treating this stuck tension. The cause of remedy is to reset and retrain the fearful device to recognize that there's no threat.

five. Take right care of signs and symptoms

Somatic treatment is beneficial for introduced than in reality humans with PTSD. It can be used to remedy lots of situations, together with:

Stress Depression

Enduring soreness

Substance use issues (SUDs) due to the fact somatic experiencing specializes in frame sensations and emotional tool management, it can teach people higher techniques to suppose and help rewire the mind to create a healthful stability.

This shape of treatment will boom human beings's hobby of their intellectual reports, which include emotions and sensations. By using each top-down and backside-up techniques, individuals can benefit a deeper expertise of the way their our our bodies respond to trauma and the way to do away with it.

Chapter 14: Polyvagas Theory And The Vagus Nerves

A new psychology take a look at is asking at Poly Vagal Theory and the feature of the vagus nerve in making us experience secure. According to Jill Miller, "that may be a manner to talk for your senses—your feelings, your urges, and your frame's wishes—in a aware manner."

People knew the most approximately the nervous tool in dimensions before to Poly Vagal Theory. The sympathetic response is our "fight or flight" reaction, whereas the parasympathetic reaction is our "freeze or faint" response. More activation equals greater arousal in this -way precept, on the equal time as lots much less activation equals less arousal. However, the start of Poly Vagal Theory takes a far much less black-and-white technique. As a surrender end result, it consists of a 3rd response that each awakens and settles down. How? Poly Vagal Theory investigates the vagus nerve and its capabilities.

The Vagus Nerve

The vagus nerve connects the brain to numerous important organs in the body, which encompass the intestine, coronary coronary coronary heart, and lungs. The Latin term for "wandering" is wherein the word "vagus" originates from. As a give up end result, the vagus nerve "wanders" to other areas of the body. The vagus nerve is cut up into quantities, one within the all over again and one within the the the front. The dorsal branch results within the top of our frame (to our 1/three eye), whilst the ventral branch ends in the lowest (to our 0.33 eye). However, the dorsal and ventral branches of the vagus nerve feature mainly strategies.

The unmyelinated vagus nerve or the dorsal branch of the vagus nerve leads the body to shut down. By "locating out," the body defends itself from the effects of stressful reviews.

However, on the identical time as this can assist within the initial case of trauma, it does now not assist as loads if we stay in this country. This is why the ventral department of the vagus nerve, furthermore called the myelinated vagus nerve, is so crucial.

This is as it does no longer surely close to down the frame, however as an alternative attempts to repair normalcy.

Exercise #1

Squats

Strength education is important. The extra muscle health you have got got had been given, the more electricity you can burn.

This is energy sporting events and it labored on more than one muscle institution. Squats are an tremendous instance due to the truth they paintings the quads, hamstrings, and gluteals.

You get the maximum in your cash with them because of the fact they art work the maximum muscle businesses right now. Form is probably very crucial.

What makes an hobby beneficial is how it's miles performed. It's no longer beneficial if you do no longer do it proper.

Keep proper form through retaining your toes shoulder-width apart and your again right now.

Drop your lower back and bend your knees. As a good buy as viable, the knee want to be close to the ankle.

Think approximately how you'll sit down down in a chair if it wasn't there.

Start thru getting right at stepping into and out of a real chair. Once you could do that, strive tapping your bottom on the chair and then getting up. Then do it yet again, however this time without the chair.

Many people whinge of knee pain, it absolutely is regularly because of inclined quads. If it hurts to stroll down the stairs, do squats to bolster your legs.

Exercise #2

Lunges, like squats, work all of the critical lower-frame muscle mass, together with the gluteals, quads, and hamstrings.

A lunge is a great technique to exercising session due to the reality it's far much like on foot but a good buy greater hard.

Lunges are a complicated form of squats that still help you enhance your balance.

Here's the way you need to pass about it:

Take a large breakthrough on the same time as preserving a without delay decrease returned. Maintain your weight for your decrease again ft and reduce your lower once more leg's knee closer to the ground whilst bending your front knee to round 90 ranges.

You keep in mind sitting for your rear foot, however the leg on which you ought to take a seat is the most effective behind you.

To make a lunge extra useful, bear in mind going backward and forward further to ahead and backward.

Chapter 15: Energy Psychology

The quite cutting-edge challenge of electricity psychology is a department of integrative medicinal drug that combines Eastern views at the mind and frame with Western theories of psychology and psychotherapy. According to proponents of energy psychotherapy, treating anxiety troubles, phobias, and positioned up-disturbing pressure ailment (PTSD) thru tapping on acupuncture websites on the identical time as considering a few factor that motives worry can be beneficial.

Research that is nonetheless being finished shows that this remedy, no matter the truth that it is despite the fact that clearly debatable, might be a promising treatment.

In the early Nineteen Eighties, Roger Callahan, PhD, popularised energy psychology remedies underneath the identify of "idea location remedy." David Feinstein, PhD, a medical psychologist, is the writer of an energy psychology training direction that is supplied to both highbrow fitness experts and non-experts alike.

Types of Energy Psychology

The time period "energy psychology" refers to a preference of numerous healing techniques. Some examples are:

Emotional Freedom Technique (EFT)

EFT is a form of energy psychology wherein disturbing-inducing recollections are paired with tapping focused spots at the body in addition to using verbal affirmations. This manner is called the Emotional Freedom Technique (EFT). This treatment can each be completed inside the affected person's domestic by means of way of themselves or through a licensed therapist.

Thought Field Therapy (TFT)

Is a shape of energy psychology that includes tapping on severa regions of the frame in a predetermined collection. These sequences are decided using quite a few strategies, each of which became advanced to deal with a specific subject. Tapping is utilized in each belief challenge remedy and EFT. In concept subject remedy, tapping is blended with a painful, difficult, or worrying memory. These steps can be accomplished through a skilled therapist, however the therapy additionally can be observed out and finished on one's very own thru every body who's worried.

Tapas Acupressure Therapy (TAT)

It's a way created with the useful resource of acupuncturists in which pressure is applied with the hands to precise locations at the pinnacle and face. While using this strain, people go through a series of thoughts that target the reasons in their troubles, the causes of their modern-day difficulties, powerful imagery, and in the end, forgiveness and healing. As is the case with other sub-fields of strength psychology, this sub-problem can each be practised at domestic or via an expert practitioner who has obtained formal education.

Benefits of Energy Psychology

There are a multitude of blessings to strength psychology, which may additionally make it an appealing healing desire.

Listed below are some of the blessings

Accessibility

Due to the gain with which they may be positioned, the strategies of power psychology can be practised and taught via a massive style of clinical and intellectual fitness practitioners, which incorporates however no longer limited to physicians, psychologists, therapists, counsellors, and holistic healers.

Approach and Simplicity

The truth that a whole lot of those techniques can be learnt and practiced in the convenience of one's non-public domestic makes this a superb preference for oldsters which is probably searching out strategies that can be incorporated into normal lifestyles.

Low Risk

Techniques from the field of strength psychology that contain a low danger seem like secure and may be of use in enjoyable. Some proponents have characterized it as having maximum of the equal benefits as acupuncture, but without the use of needles, that may be a exquisite difference from conventional acupuncture.